THE

PCOS

DIET COOKBOOK

365 Days of Delicious Recipes to Nourish and Regulate

Hormones, Manage PCOS Symptoms, and Empower

Girls on their Journey to Hormonal Balance

OLIVIA THOMPSON

TABLE OF CONTENTS

INTRODUCTION

Welcome to *The PCOS Diet Cookbook*, your comprehensive guide to managing Polycystic Ovary Syndrome (PCOS) through nutrition and lifestyle changes. I am Olivia Thompson, a devoted nutritionist who holds a special interest in women's health and possesses a profound comprehension of the obstacles experienced by those with PCOS. Throughout my journey, I have seen how food can remarkably transform health and wellness, and it fuels my passion for helping individuals in their pursuit of well-being. I believe that an excellent diet is not just about preventing deficiencies but about establishing the optimum intake of food components to promote health and reduce the risk of diseases. This outlook is the core of my profession and this recipe collection. In recent years, our comprehension of how food contributes to human health has profoundly transformed. We now know that a balanced diet is key to not just improving life expectancy but also enhancing life quality. This book is a testament to this understanding, offering you a roadmap to an excellent nutrition plan designed specifically for managing PCOS.

The PCOS Diet Cookbook is not just a collection of recipes; it's a tool to empower you on your journey to hormonal balance. It aims to educate you about PCOS, its causes, symptoms, and treatment options and inspire you to take charge of your health. The book provides practical advice on meal planning, portion control, and long-term dietary strategies, emphasizing the importance of sustainable lifestyle changes for effective PCOS management.

The recipes in this book are delicious, nourishing, and specifically designed to support hormonal balance and manage PCOS symptoms. They incorporate nutrient-dense ingredients and balance macronutrients to provide nourishment and promote overall well-being.

In addition to the recipes, you will find comprehensive information about PCOS, practical advice on meal planning, and tips for long-term success. The book also includes lifestyle tips for hormonal balance, such as exercise recommendations, stress management techniques, sleep optimization strategies, and self-care practices.

The primary objective of this book is to convey that a PCOS diagnosis isn't an irreversible verdict, but rather a catalyst for change. It's an opportunity to take control of your health, embrace nourishing food, and make sustainable lifestyle changes that will help you live a vibrant, fulfilling life.

I invite you to embark on this journey of wellness with me. Let's navigate the path to hormonal balance together, using food as our ally. Always keep in mind that you're not alone on this path, and with appropriate resources and information, you can flourish despite having PCOS.

Welcome to a universe of delectable and nutritious meals that bolster your overall health and wellness.

CHAPTER 1

UNDERSTANDING PCOS: CAUSES, SYMPTOMS, AND TREATMENT OPTIONS

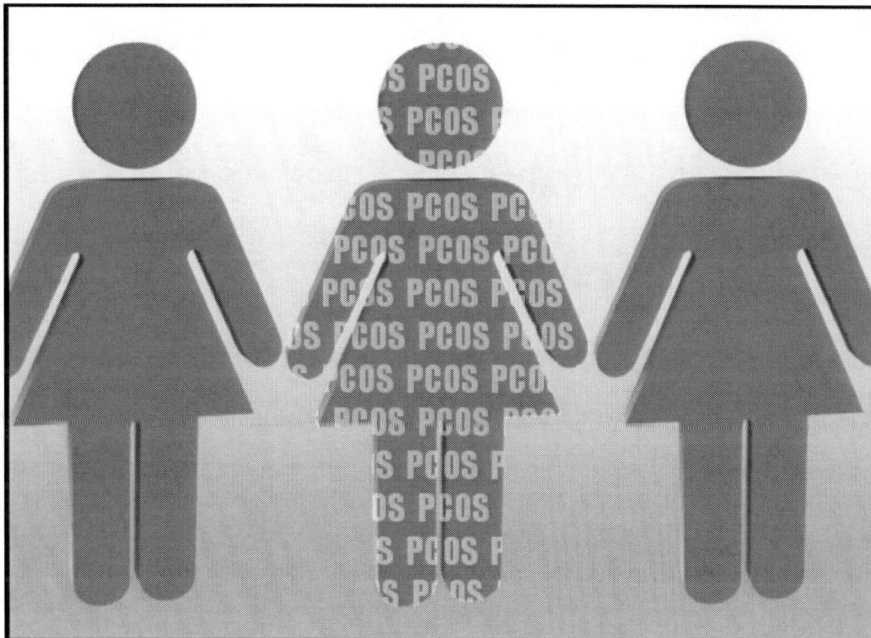

Polycystic Ovary Syndrome, commonly known as PCOS, is a prevalent endocrine disorder that affects millions of women worldwide. First recognized in the 1930s, PCOS remains a significant health concern in contemporary society. This comprehensive section aims to provide readers with an in-depth understanding of PCOS, shedding light on its causes, symptoms, and various treatment options available.

WHAT IS PCOS?

Polycystic ovary syndrome (PCOS) is a medical condition characterized by the excessive production of androgens, which are male sex hormones typically found in small quantities in women. Polycystic ovary syndrome, often referred to as PCOS is a medical condition distinguished by the existence of numerous tiny cysts or fluid-filled pouches within the ovaries. However, it is important to note that not all women with this illness produce cysts, and conversely, some women without the disorder may still develop cysts. Ovulation refers to the process of the release of a mature egg from an ovary. This happens to enable male sperm to fertilize it. During your menstrual cycle, if the egg is not fertilized, it is expelled from the body through menstruation.

In certain rare situations, a woman may experience insufficient production of the hormones necessary for ovulation. When ovulation does not occur, it can lead to the development of numerous small cysts in the ovaries. These cysts produce hormones called androgens. Females diagnosed with polycystic ovary syndrome (PCOS) frequently exhibit elevated quantities of androgen hormones. This can worsen the difficulties experienced during a woman's menstrual cycle. It can also cause many of the symptoms commonly associated with PCOS. PCOS is often treated with medication. While it doesn't provide a definitive cure for PCOS, it can aid in relieving symptoms and decreasing the likelihood of associated health complications.

What Is the Root Cause of PCOS?

The exact origin of PCOS remains uncertain. It is observed that many women with PCOS exhibit insulin resistance, meaning their bodies struggle to use insulin efficiently. The body experiences an increase in insulin levels, which can potentially result in elevated androgen levels. In addition, obesity can increase insulin levels, which can worsen the symptoms of PCOS. Polycystic ovary syndrome (PCOS) has a tendency to be hereditary. Polycystic ovary syndrome (PCOS) commonly occurs among sisters, mothers, and daughters.

What Are the Dangers of PCOS?

There's a higher likelihood of you having PCOS if it's a condition that your mother or sister has been diagnosed with. Furthermore, the prevalence increases in those who struggle with insulin resistance or obesity.

COMMON SYMPTOMS OF PCOS

PCOS manifests through a range of symptoms, which include:

- Excessive body hair growth (hirsutism), especially noticeable on parts of the body like the face, chest, and back.
- Difficulties in achieving pregnancy (infertility).
- Presence of numerous or large-sized cysts in the ovaries.
- Thinning of hair or hair loss in a pattern similar to male-pattern baldness.
- Oily skin or frequent breakouts of acne.
- Dark or thick patches of skin on the back of the neck, under the arms, or across the chest.
- Irregular menstrual cycles, which could be infrequent, very light, or completely absent.
- Small growths of skin, known as skin tags, located in the armpits or neck.
- Weight gain, often concentrated around the abdominal area.

DIAGNOSING PCOS

The identification of polycystic ovary syndrome (PCOS) is not possible with a single test. Your doctor will most likely start by asking about how you're feeling, what drugs you're taking, and if you have any other health concerns. Your doctor may also be interested in learning about your weight and menstrual cycle history. Increased hair growth, resistance to insulin, and acne will all be factors in a physical examination. Then, your doctor may suggest that you:

- Pelvic examination. Any abnormalities in your reproductive organs might prompt your doctor to do a pelvic check.
- Blood tests are carried out. Blood tests can detect hormone concentrations. Menstrual abnormalities and PCOS mimics, including androgen excesses, can both be diagnosed and treated with the use of this tests. Diagnostics of fasting triglyceride and cholesterol levels in the blood may also be taken. The way your body handles sugar (glucose) is measured by taking a glucose tolerance test.
- Ultrasound. Your ovarian appearance and uterine lining thickness can both be evaluated with an ultrasound. A transducer, which looks like a wand, is placed into your vagina. The sound waves generated by the transducer are converted into on-screen representations through a digital processor.

Your doctor may suggest further testing to rule out other conditions if you've been diagnosed with polycystic ovarian syndrome (PCOS). The levels of glucose tolerance, blood pressure, cholesterol, and triglycerides should be monitored routinely. Anxiety and depression screening, in addition to sleep apnea assessment.

TREATMENT APPROACHES FOR PCOS

The management of PCOS is affected by a number of variables. Your age, the intensity of your symptoms, and your general health may all play a role. Your treatment options may be affected by your future fertility goals.

If you do decide to become pregnant, your therapy may involve the following:

- Implementing changes in nutrition and physical activity. In order to lose weight and alleviate your symptoms, it is beneficial to adopt a nutritious diet and engage in regular physical activity. In addition, they have the potential to enhance insulin utilization, reduce blood glucose levels, and potentially promote ovulation.
- Ovulation-inducing medications are used to stimulate ovulation. Medications can help stimulate regular egg production in the ovaries. These drugs carry risks and should not be taken lightly. They can increase the chances of having multiple children, such as twins or more. Ovarian hyperstimulation may also be caused by them. This condition occurs when the ovaries generate an excessive amount of hormones. Symptoms that may occur include abdominal bloating and pelvic pain.

The following interventions may be included in your treatment plan if you do not wish to conceive:

- Pills for birth control: This helps with a few things: regular periods, lower testosterone, and less breakouts.
- Treatment for diabetes. This treatment is commonly used to address insulin resistance in individuals with PCOS. Additionally, it can potentially reduce testosterone levels, restrict hair growth, and promote more frequent ovulation.
- Improving nutrition and increasing physical activity. In order to lose weight and alleviate your symptoms, it is important to maintain a nutritious diet and engage in regular physical activity. In addition, they have the potential to enhance insulin utilization efficiency, reduce blood glucose levels, and potentially promote ovulation.

Aside from lifestyle changes, certain medications may also be employed to manage other symptoms. For instance, specific drugs can help reduce hair growth and improve skin conditions such as acne. Your healthcare provider might recommend the following strategies to control excessive hair growth and alleviate acne:

- Spironolactone (Aldactone): This medication acts to inhibit the effects of androgens on the skin, which includes issues like excessive hair growth and acne. Given the risk of birth defects associated with Spironolactone, it's crucial to ensure reliable birth control is used while taking this medication. It is not recommended for those who are pregnant or planning to conceive.
- Eflornithine (Vaniqa): This is a topical cream that can assist in slowing the growth of facial hair.
- Hair Removal Procedures: These involve methods like electrolysis and laser hair removal. In the electrolysis process, a tiny needle is inserted into each individual hair follicle, which then emits an electrical current. This energy first damages, then destroys the follicle. Laser hair removal is a medical procedure that effectively removes undesired hair by using an intense beam of light.
- You may require numerous electrolysis or laser hair removal sessions. Other choices include shaving, plucking, or applying treatments that destroy unwanted hair. However, these are only temporary, and the hair may thicken as it comes back.
- Treatments for acne; acne medications, such as tablets and topical creams or gels, may help. Consult your doctor about your options.

THE ROLE OF DIET IN MANAGING PCOS

The 2018 PCOS guideline acknowledges that there is inadequate data to show that any specific dietary choices improve health outcomes. As per general population recommendations, dietary recommendations may include a number of balanced dietary methods according to the individual's lifestyle demands and preferences.

This advice stems from a comprehensive review which compared various dietary approaches (for instance, low carbohydrate, low GI and GL, high protein, diets enriched with MUFA, and fat-counting diets) for optimal PCOS management. The review found only slight differences in anthropometric outcomes and concluded that weight loss enhances PCOS symptoms irrespective of the specifics of the dietary plan. A growing body of evidence suggests that a variety of dietary interventions may have beneficial effects on PCOS traits that occur independently of weight loss. It is critical that the emerging findings from these studies be thoroughly reviewed in order to promote the interests of consumers and health professionals. To summarize current information, this review divided diets into those that adjust carbs, protein, and fat, as well as those that follow specific dietary patterns.

Carbohydrates

The most investigated dietary method for PCOS therapy is the use of altered carbohydrate composition. Two systematic reviews published after the guideline's creation support adjusted carbohydrate consumption to improve intermediate markers of PCOS, concluding that changing carbohydrate type rather than content is preferable for improved PCOS management. Adhering to a diet with a low Glycemic Index (GI) or Glycemic Load (GL) for a minimum of eight weeks significantly decreases Waist Circumference (WC) and Body Mass Index (BMI) compared to a high GI/GL or standard diet. However, the amount of weight loss is usually similar to that observed with other dietary compositions. These reductions are claimed to be the result of decreased hunger, which may lower calorie consumption and make long-term dietary guidelines simpler to follow. When compared to high carbohydrate or control diets, low GI/GL diets improve insulin sensitivity and reproductive hormones (T, SHBG, FAI), contributing to improvements in reproductive function, notably monthly regularity. Finally, when compared to a regular or high-GI/GL diet, low-GI/GL diets can improve risk variables for T2DM and CVD, such as glucose, LDL-C, and HDL-C. It should be emphasized that the health benefits of low-GI and low-GL diets can also be attributable to proportional increases in protein and/or fat loading.

Protein

When compared to high-carbohydrate diets, higher protein intakes may be superior at suppressing testosterone levels in women with PCOS. Postprandial studies have demonstrated that high-protein meals can lower insulin and dehydroepiandrosterone stimulation when compared to glucose-rich meals. Reduced hunger and energy intakes from low-GI/GL diets have also been linked to higher protein intakes in the general population. High protein diets (defined here as protein containing 25% of total calories) consumed for at least four weeks lower weight, BMI, WC, WHR, and fat mass. Improved FINS and HOMA-IR, blood lipids, and hirsutism

(Ferriman-Gallwey score) are associated with these anthropometric decreases. Only three of these trials, however, were able to demonstrate statistically significant increases in anthropometric measurements, insulin sensitivity, and blood lipids when compared to low or standard protein or control diets. Only one study looked at the effects on mental health outcomes and discovered that eating more protein reduced depression and enhanced self-esteem.

Fats

Increased MUFA and polyunsaturated fatty acid (PUFA) consumption can help with metabolic problems linked with PCOS. Postprandial studies in PCOS found that high-fat meals had longer T decreases than low-fat meals, owing to delayed nutrient absorption. Two acute meal investigations in lean and obese women with and without PCOS found that proatherogenic inflammatory markers and oxidative stress were enhanced following saturated fat ingestion, independent of but augmented by obesity, with this related to worsening IR and androgens. Two studies in PCOS looked at the effects of habitual walnut (PUFA-rich diet) and almond (MUFA-rich diet) intake for at least six weeks and found no differences in glucoregulatory status, lipids, or androgens, with the exception of HbA1c being significantly lower in the walnut group compared to the almond group. Kasim-Karakas et al. found that increased walnut intake raised fasting and postprandial glucose (oral glucose tolerance test (OGTT)) compared to habitual (control), which they hypothesized was due to the control diet's high oleic acid content. These findings imply that there is little benefit to increasing dietary PUFA content when compared to MUFA levels. Two randomized controlled trials in women with PCOS looked at the effects of diets high in olive, canola, and sunflower oil. When compared to 25 g/day olive and sunflower oils, Yahay et al. found that 25 g/day canola oil reduced TAG, TC/HDL-C, LDL-C/HDL-C, TAG/HDL-C, and HOMA but not androgens. This may be due to canola oil's superior fatty acid profile, which includes comparable MUFA content to olive oil, higher alpha-linolenic acid, a lower omega-6/omega-3 ratio, and less saturated fat than both olive and sunflower oils. In a study by Douglas et al., it was observed that a balanced low-carbohydrate diet resulted in reduced weight and improved insulin response (during an oral glucose tolerance test) as compared to a diet enriched with monounsaturated fatty acids (MUFA) from olive oil. This suggests that consuming fewer carbohydrates might have a stronger impact on glucose regulation than increasing MUFA intake. In two separate randomized controlled trials, low-fat diets were compared with low-carbohydrate or low GI diets. Both types of diets resulted in reductions in weight, waist circumference, and body fat, along with improved fasting insulin levels and free androgen index. However, no significant differences were observed between the two groups.

Dietary and Eating Habits

Aside from diets that focus on specific macronutrient alterations, a variety of dietary patterns have been investigated in PCOS therapy. The Dietary Approaches to Stop Hypertension (DASH) diet, which is high in fruit, vegetables, whole grains, nuts, legumes, and low-fat dairy and has a mostly low-GI carbohydrate profile, was found to be the best choice for reducing IR in a systematic review that included 19 studies and 1,193 participants and was published after the guidelines were made (2020). Following a span of 8-12 weeks, Randomized Controlled Trials (RCTs) involving individuals with PCOS have noted advantageous outcomes concerning weight, BMI, insulin resistance (IR), and a variety of hormones, including Sex Hormone Binding Globulin (SHBG), androstenedione, and Free Androgen Index (FAI), when adhering to a Dietary Approaches to Stop Hypertension (DASH) as opposed to a regular diet. Furthermore, diets free from animal products or vegetarian diets have been found to decrease inflammation indicators such as C-reactive Protein (CRP), resistin, and adiponectin when contrasted with diets containing meat. While a completely plant-based or vegan diet led to weight reduction after three months, the results were not evident after six months. Finally, a diet centering on legumes or pulses exhibited similar effects as a generally healthy diet in terms of weight loss, enhancement of insulin sensitivity, and reduction in reproductive hormones. All of these dietary patterns are high in fiber and plant proteins, which promote microbial diversity and the generation of short-chain fatty acids with anti-inflammatory properties. Considering the evidence from mechanistic animal research suggesting a pathophysiological role for gut microbiota in IR and ovarian dysfunction, it is plausible that the metabolic and hormonal benefits related to plant-based diets in PCOS are linked to higher intakes of dietary prebiotics. More mechanistic research on the function of gut microbiota in PCOS, as well as RCTs on the impact of dietary prebiotics on PCOS outcomes, is needed.

Research has shown that adopting certain eating patterns can have positive effects on insulin sensitivity and reducing androgen levels. For example, consuming smaller, more frequent meals throughout the day and having a larger breakfast followed by a smaller dinner have been found to be beneficial. This is a significant discovery because women with PCOS are more likely to miss breakfast or eat breakfast and lunch later in the day.

Specific food items studied in relation to PCOS outcomes, such as raw onions, concentrated pomegranate juice, and flaxseed powder, have generated mostly conflicting results. One major disadvantage of these single-food studies is that foods are never taken alone within the diet, ignoring the influence of the dietary matrix and the interactions that occur between dietary constituents throughout meals. These studies have little application in terms of developing realistic dietary recommendations.

CHAPTER 2

THE PCOS DIET: BASICS AND GUIDELINES

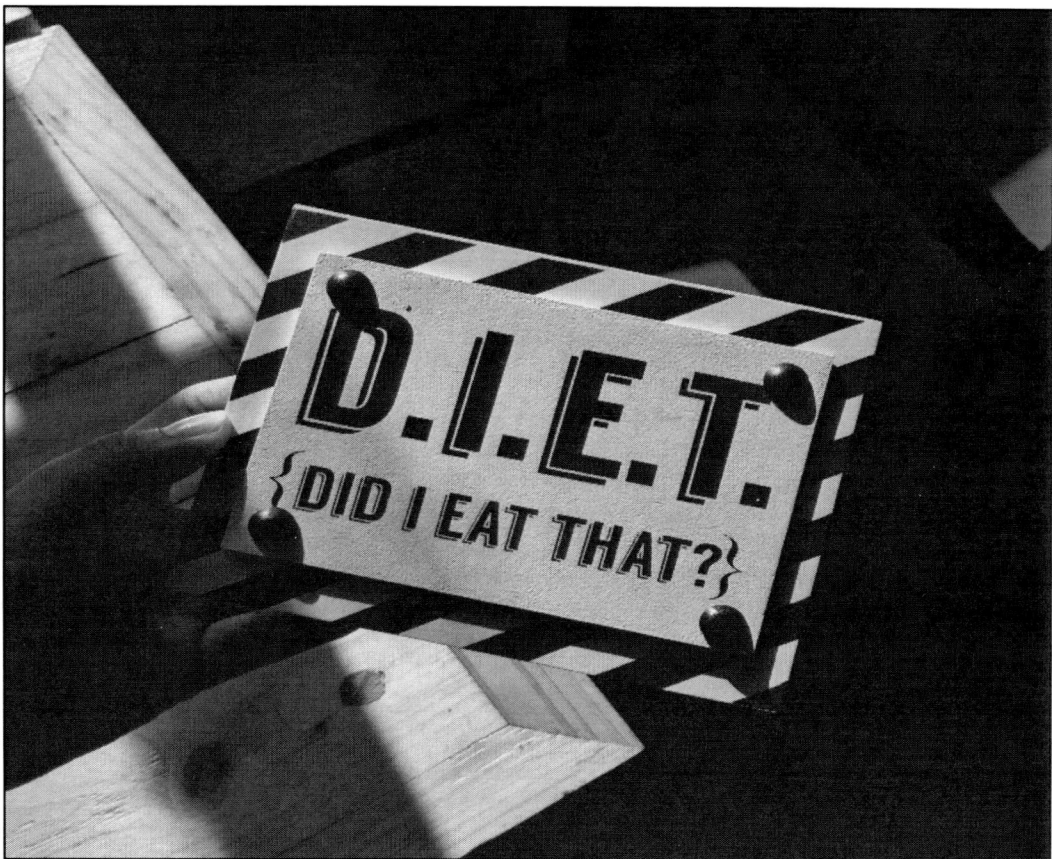

A critical component in managing PCOS is the adoption of a healthy lifestyle, encompassing a balanced and thoughtfully constructed eating plan. In this section, we will investigate the role of nutrition in handling PCOS and examine the essential guidelines of the PCOS diet. Moreover, we will discuss the specific foods that should be included or avoided in this dietary approach, along with the importance of meal planning and portion control. Lastly, we will provide valuable strategies to ensure long-term success in adhering to the PCOS diet.

THE IMPORTANCE OF NUTRITION IN PCOS MANAGEMENT

Appropriate dietary habits are of paramount importance in managing PCOS. Given that this disorder is associated with hormonal disruptions, resistance to insulin, and inflammation, the implementation of a wholesome diet can aid in symptom reduction and enhance overall health. By making the right dietary choices, women with PCOS can promote hormonal balance, enhance insulin sensitivity, and reduce inflammation, ultimately leading to better reproductive health and overall quality of life.

The PCOS diet aims to regulate insulin levels, as insulin resistance is a common issue associated with PCOS. Hormonal disruptions and PCOS symptoms are the result of insulin resistance, which causes the body to produce more androgens. A well-designed PCOS diet can help manage insulin resistance and minimize its impact on the body, thereby improving fertility and lowering the risk of long-term consequences such as type 2 diabetes and cardiovascular disease.

KEY PRINCIPLES OF THE PCOS DIET

The Polycystic Ovary Syndrome (PCOS) diet is not just a diet; it's a lifestyle approach designed to manage the symptoms of PCOS and promote hormonal balance. It's based on scientific research and clinical experience, and it emphasizes the importance of nutrient-dense foods, balanced macronutrients, and sustainable lifestyle changes. Here are the key principles of the PCOS diet:

1. Equilibrium of Macronutrients: The dietary approach to PCOS underlines the significance of maintaining a balance among macronutrients - proteins, carbohydrates, and fats. Each of these macronutrients holds an essential role in maintaining hormonal equilibrium and overall health.
   - Carbohydrates: Choose healthy vegetables, fruits, and grains over simple carbs such as white bread, spaghetti, and sugary snacks. Complex carbohydrates undergo a slow digestion process, aiding in the stability of blood glucose levels, a vital aspect in the control of PCOS.
   - Proteins: Include lean proteins in your diet, such as fish, poultry, tofu, and legumes. Proteins are essential for hormone production and can help control blood sugar levels.

- Fats: Focus on healthy fats, such as avocados, nuts, seeds, and olive oil. These fats are essential for hormone production and can help reduce inflammation, a common issue in women with PCOS.

2. High Fiber Intake: A fiber-rich diet can help treat PCOS by delaying digestion and lowering the impact of sugar on the blood, hence aiding in blood sugar regulation. Consume lots of fruits, veggies, whole grains, and legumes.

3. Anti-Inflammatory Foods: PCOS is often linked with low-grade inflammation. Including anti-inflammatory food items such as berries, oily fish, leafy green veggies, and extra virgin olive oil in your diet can aid in controlling this inflammation.

4. Consistent Dietary Schedule: Consuming food at regular intervals can aid in keeping blood sugar and insulin levels stable, a key factor in managing PCOS. Ensure that each meal and snack includes a mix of protein, fats, and carbohydrates.

5. Minimize Intake of Refined Foods and Sugars: The consumption of refined foods and sugars can result in blood sugar and insulin spikes, worsening the symptoms of PCOS. Try to reduce your consumption of such foods, sweetened beverages, and snacks high in sugar.

6. Ensure Proper Hydration: Keeping yourself well-hydrated is vital for overall well-being and can also help in dealing with PCOS symptoms. The goal should be to drink at least 8 glasses of water per day, and even more, if you are physically active or living in a warmer environment.

7. Conscious Consumption: Be aware of your body's signals for hunger and satiety. Engaging in mindful eating can assist you in understanding your body's requirements and avoid overconsumption of food.

Bear in mind, the PCOS diet does not adhere to a 'one solution fits all' method. It's a set of guidelines which can be customized to suit your unique needs, preferences, and way of life. Always engage in a discussion with a healthcare professional or a certified dietitian before implementing significant alterations to your eating habits.

The goal of the PCOS diet is to support hormonal balance, manage symptoms, and improve your overall quality of life. It's about nourishing your body with the nutrients it needs to thrive, not depriving or restricting yourself. With the right approach, the PCOS diet can be a delicious, satisfying, and sustainable way to manage PCOS.

FOODS TO INCLUDE AND AVOID

Foods to Include

1. Fruits and Vegetables: Incorporate a diverse array of colorful fruits and vegetables into the diet. These foods, abundant in nutrients, supply vital vitamins, minerals, and antioxidants that assist in managing hormones and combating inflammation.
2. Lean Proteins: Opt for sources of protein that are low in fat, like poultry without skin, seafood, lean meats, tofu, and beans. Protein is essential for tissue repair and plays a role in hormone synthesis.
3. Whole Grains: Select whole grain options such as brown rice, oatmeal, quinoa, and whole wheat bread, which provide complex carbohydrates and fiber, essential for maintaining consistent blood sugar levels and supporting digestive health.
4. Beneficial Fats: Incorporate food items high in beneficial fats like nuts, seeds, avocados, and olive oil in your meals. These fats support hormone production and can reduce inflammation.
5. Dairy Alternatives: For those with lactose intolerance or sensitivity, dairy alternatives like almond milk or soy milk can be excellent choices.

Foods to Avoid

1. High Glycemic Index Foods: Minimize or avoid high GI foods like sugary beverages, white bread, pastries, and sweets, as they can cause rapid spikes in blood sugar levels and worsen insulin resistance.
2. Processed Foods: Stay away from heavily processed foods, as they often contain unhealthy fats, added sugars, and artificial additives that can aggravate inflammation and contribute to weight gain.
3. Saturated and Trans Fats: Aim to lower your intake of saturated fats, which are typically present in red meat, butter, and high-fat dairy products, as well as trans fats often found in processed snacks and deep-fried items.
4. Caffeine and Alcohol: Although moderate consumption of caffeine and alcohol might not pose significant harm, overconsumption could disrupt hormonal equilibrium and affect sleep cycles, posing challenges for managing PCOS effectively.

MEAL PLANNING AND PORTION CONTROL

Meal Planning

Meal planning is a fundamental aspect of the PCOS diet that involves carefully selecting and organizing meals and snacks to ensure balanced nutrition and adherence to dietary guidelines. Effective meal planning can help individuals with PCOS maintain steady blood sugar levels, manage weight, and support hormonal balance. Here are some key steps and considerations for successful meal planning:

1. Set Goals and Create a Weekly Menu: Start by setting specific dietary goals based on individual health needs and preferences. Subsequently, develop a weekly meal plan that incorporates a diverse array of foods abundant in nutrients from various food groups. Strive for a combination of fruits, lean proteins, whole grains, vegetables, and beneficial fats.

2. Integrate a Spectrum of Fruits and Vegetables: Add a diverse array of vibrant fruits and vegetables into your meal plan. Different colors indicate varying nutrients and antioxidants that support overall health and help combat inflammation. Consider seasonal produce for variety and cost-effectiveness.

3. Batch Cooking and Preparing Ahead: Batch cooking is a time-saving strategy where larger quantities of meals are prepared at once and stored for future consumption. This can be especially beneficial for busy days when there is limited time for cooking. Divide the Meals into Single Servings: Separate the prepared dishes into individual portions and keep them in the fridge or freezer for convenience.

4. Ensure Balanced Macronutrient Distribution: Aim for each meal to include a proportionate amount of macronutrients – carbs, proteins, and fats. For example, a well-balanced dinner might include a serving of grilled chicken (protein), quinoa (carbohydrate), and a side of roasted vegetables drizzled with olive oil (healthy fat).

5. Mindful Snacking: Plan for healthy snacks that can curb hunger and prevent overeating during mealtimes. Nuts, seeds, Greek yogurt, and fresh fruit are excellent choices for satisfying and nutrient-dense snacks.

6. Scrutinize Food Labels and Minimize Processed Foods: In your meal planning, pay attention to food labels to spot processed items that are high in added sugars, unhealthy fats, and synthetic additives. Reduce or exclude these from your plan as they can exacerbate insulin resistance and inflammation.

7. Stay Hydrated: Hydration is also key. Water is vital for comprehensive health and aids in managing weight. Try to consume ample amounts of water during the day, and for an extra twist, consider infusing it with fresh fruits or herbs.

Portion Control

Portion control refers to the act of managing the quantity of food intake during meals and snack times. It is an essential strategy for weight management and preventing overeating, which can exacerbate insulin resistance and PCOS symptoms. Here are some effective methods to master portion control in your daily life:

1. Choose Lesser-Sized Dishware: Using plates and bowls of a smaller size can visually help keep your portions in check. Since we have a tendency to load up our plates irrespective of their size, smaller dishware can subconsciously guide us towards smaller serving sizes.

2. Follow Serving Size Recommendations: Familiarize yourself with serving size recommendations on food labels. A great deal of pre-packaged food products offer details about the recommended portion size as well as the total number of servings within each package. Adhering to these suggestions can help prevent inadvertent overconsumption.

3. Listen to Your Body: Pay attention to hunger and fullness cues while eating. Eating slowly and mindfully can help you recognize when you are satisfied, preventing you from consuming more food than your body needs.

4. Distribute Snacks Evenly: Refrain from munching directly from sizeable snack packets, which can make it tricky to monitor your intake. Rather, divide your snacks into distinct portions to better manage your consumption.

5. Opt for Non-Starchy Veggies: Vegetables that aren't high in starch are beneficial as they contain fewer calories and a high amount of fiber. This makes them perfect for serving large portions without worrying about exceeding your calorie limit. Prioritize vegetables as a substantial portion of your meal.

6. Measure Portions Initially: If you are unsure about appropriate portion sizes, use measuring cups and scales to measure food quantities until you develop a better sense of proper portions.

7. Refrain from Screen-Time Eating: Consuming food while engaged in a TV show or computer work can encourage unconscious overconsumption. Instead, center your attention on your meal, relishing the taste and feel of the food.

STRATEGIES FOR LONG-TERM SUCCESS

While adopting the PCOS diet can bring about positive changes in the management of Polycystic Ovary Syndrome, maintaining this dietary approach over the long term can be challenging. However, with the right mindset, support, and strategies, individuals with PCOS can successfully integrate the PCOS diet into their lifestyle and experience lasting benefits. Here are some effective strategies for long-term success:

Meal Planning

Just as a builder wouldn't start construction without a blueprint, you shouldn't start your day without a meal plan. Charting out your meals ahead of time can be a significant turning point in handling PCOS effectively. It allows you to ensure that each meal is balanced with the right macronutrients - complex carbohydrates for sustained energy, lean proteins for hormone production and muscle repair, and healthy fats for inflammation control and hormone health. Start by sketching out a simple plan for the week. Remember, the goal is not to create a gourmet menu but to ensure you have a roadmap to guide your nutritional intake.

Cook at Home

The charm of home-cooking lies in the fact that it lets you be in charge of your culinary space. You decide what goes into your dishes, how they are prepared, and how much is served. This control is vital when managing PCOS as it allows you to limit processed foods and ensure your meals are nutrient-dense. Experiment with different recipes from this book, play with spices and herbs and discover the joy of creating meals that nourish your body and tantalize your taste buds.

Mindful Eating

In our fast-paced world, it's easy to eat while distracted - in front of the TV, at our desks, or on the go. However, this can lead to overeating and a disconnection from our body's hunger and fullness cues. Mindful eating involves fully focusing on the act of consuming food, cherishing each mouthful, and acknowledging your body's cues. It centers around establishing a balanced connection with food, perceiving it as a means of nourishment rather than a source of solace or anxiety.

Regular Exercise

Physical activity is a crucial part of managing PCOS. It helps to improve insulin sensitivity, manage weight, and reduce stress levels. However, this doesn't imply that you have to dedicate long hours to rigorous gym workouts. Seek out a form of physical activity that brings you pleasure, such as dancing, hiking, practicing yoga, or engaging in gardening. The objective is to engage in movement that not only brings you happiness but also seamlessly integrates into your everyday routine.

Stress Management

Stress is like a silent saboteur when it comes to managing PCOS. Elevated stress levels can intensify symptoms and impede your ability to adhere to your dietary and physical activity plans. Therefore, incorporating strategies to handle stress into your daily schedule can be advantageous. These could range from deep breathing exercises and yoga, to keeping a journal or allocating time to commune with nature. Identify what strategy suits you best and make it an unalterable element of your everyday regime.

Adequate Sleep

Sleep is not just a leisurely activity; it's an essential component of our health. Our bodies rejuvenate, heal, and restore during sleep, which includes the harmonization of our hormones. Insufficient sleep can disrupt this harmony and exacerbate the symptoms of PCOS. Strive to obtain between 7 and 9 hours of quality sleep every night. Construct an environment conducive to sleep - dark, serene, and cool - and form a tranquil routine before bedtime to convey to your body that it's time to rest.

Regular Check-ups

Consider the approach you'd take with regular maintenance of your vehicle - this is how you should view routine visits with your healthcare professional in terms of managing PCOS. These appointments allow you to monitor your progress, make necessary adjustments to your treatment plan, and address any emerging issues or concerns. They provide an excellent opportunity for communication and collaborative decision-making with your healthcare professional.

Support Network

The journey to managing PCOS can sometimes feel lonely, but remember, you're not alone. Connecting with others who are on a similar journey can provide emotional support, practical advice, and a sense of community. This could manifest as a local community group, a digital discussion platform, or even a circle of friends who share similar goals of pursuing a healthy lifestyle.

Patience and Self-Compassion

Transitioning your habits isn't an overnight process, and it's the same case with managing PCOS. You'll face times of progress and regression, victories and challenges. It's crucial to practice patience with yourself and rejoice in every bit of forward momentum, no matter its size. During moments of setback, extend to yourself the same empathy and compassion that you'd give to a close friend. Keep in mind this is a path of steady improvement, not absolute perfection.

Thank you for your purchase!

We extend our sincere gratitude for choosing "The PCOS Diet Cookbook"

as a part of your reading repertoire.

Scan this QR-CODE to get your **FREE BONUS BOOK** resource carefully curated

to deepen your understanding of effective love and relationship mastery,

self-care practices, and techniques for fostering lasting connections.

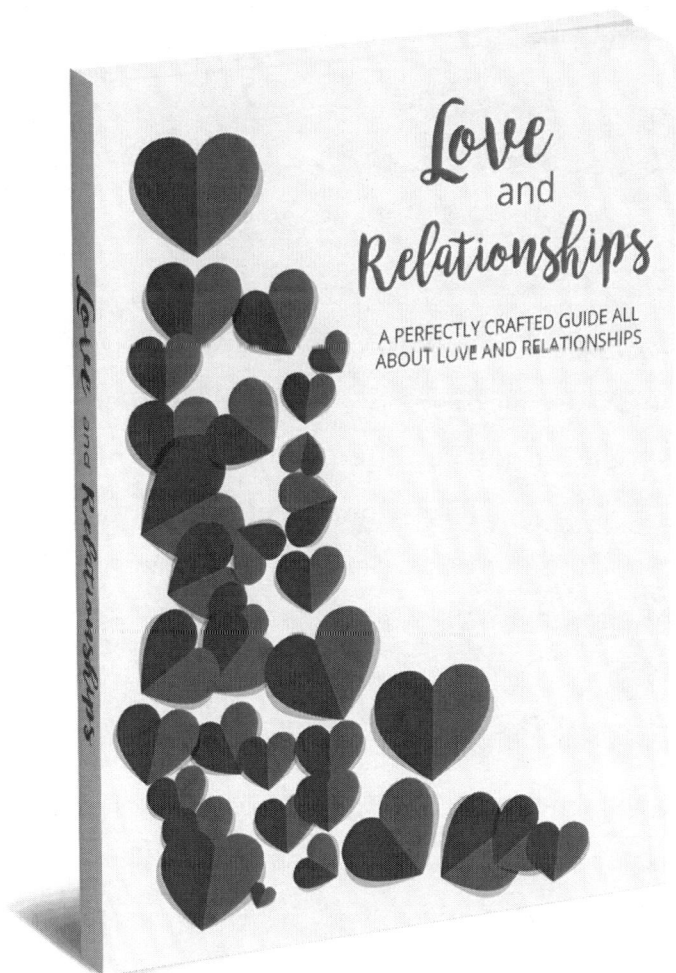

SCAN ME

CHAPTER 3

BREAKFAST DELIGHTS

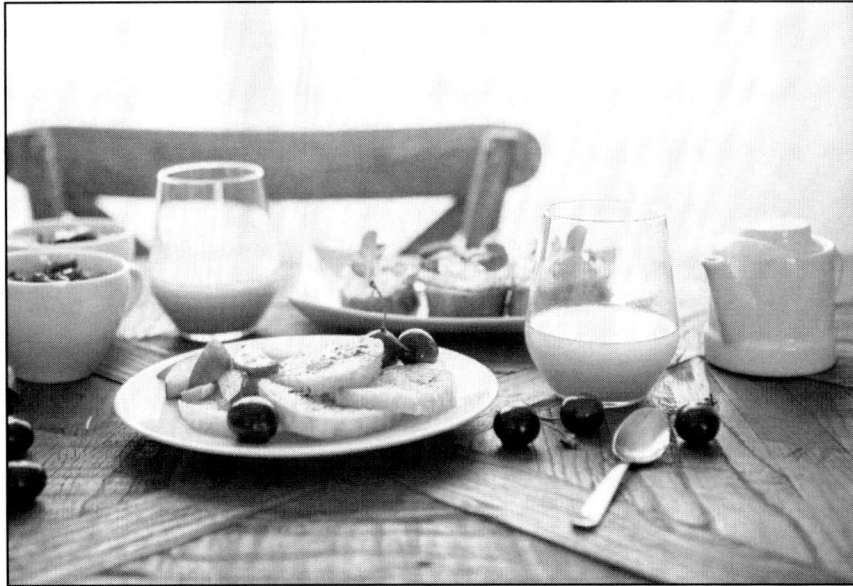

There is no one diet that is optimal for PCOS. Dietary adjustments must instead be tailored to the individual's needs, and the type of Picositos regulate blood glucose; it is best to eat a range of nutrient-dense foods, antioxidant-rich foods, and lots of protein and healthy fats. Because many PCOS women also have insulin resistance, eating plenty of protein, fats, and fiber can help balance blood glucose. Consider using peanut butter instead of syrup on your pancakes to help reduce a blood sugar surge.

Breakfast Ingredients for People With PCOS

Several nutrients are essential for PCOS management. Ideally, include as many nutrients as possible in your breakfast. However, not every meal will have every nutrient, which is fine. In fact, you might not obtain all of these in one day, which is fine. The goal with PCOS is that most meals are generally balanced. This includes a wide range of nutritional grains, proteins, healthy fats, and plant foods. According to research, there are some nutrients that may be especially beneficial for PCOS.

15 RECIPES

Powerhouse Quinoa Porridge

Prep Time:	Cook Time:	Serving Size:
5 minutes	15 minutes	2 persons

INGREDIENTS:

- 1/2 cup quinoa, rinsed
- 1 cup of non-sweetened almond milk (or any plant-based milk)
- 1 ripe banana, mashed
- 2 tablespoons almond butter
- 1 tablespoon honey or maple syrup
- 1/2 teaspoon ground cinnamon
- 1/4 teaspoon pure vanilla extract
- Fresh berries and sliced bananas for topping

INSTRUCTIONS:

- In a saucepan, combine the rinsed quinoa and almond milk. Increase the heat to medium until the mixture starts to boil.
- Lower the heat to a simmer and cover the quinoa, allowing it to cook for approximately 10-15 minutes until all the liquid is absorbed and the quinoa appears fluffy.
- Integrate the mashed banana, almond butter, honey or maple syrup, cinnamon powder, and natural vanilla extract by stirring them into the quinoa. Mix well to incorporate all the flavors.
- Divide the quinoa porridge into two serving bowls.
- Top each portion with fresh berries and sliced bananas for added nutrients and a burst of natural sweetness.
- Enjoy the powerhouse quinoa porridge as a hearty and nourishing breakfast to kickstart your day.

NUTRITIONAL FACTS (PER SERVING):

- Calories: approximately 350 kcal
- Carbohydrates: 54g
- Protein: 9g
- Fat: 12g
- Fiber: 6g

Anti-Inflammatory Turmeric Scrambled Eggs

Prep Time:	Cook Time:	Serving Size:
5 minutes	5 minutes	2 persons

INGREDIENTS:

- 4 large eggs
- 1/4 teaspoon ground turmeric
- 1/4 teaspoon ground black pepper
- Pinch of cayenne pepper (optional)
- 2 tablespoons chopped fresh parsley or cilantro
- 1 tablespoon olive oil
- Salt to taste

INSTRUCTIONS:

- In a bowl, whisk together the eggs, ground turmeric, ground black pepper, and cayenne pepper (if using) until well combined.
- Warm a non-stick frying pan over medium heat, then add the olive oil.
- Transfer the egg blend to the pan and gently stir while cooking until the eggs reach your preferred level of being scrambled and cooked.
- Garnish with freshly chopped parsley or cilantro for an extra burst of flavor and a hint of freshness.
- Season the scrambled eggs with salt to taste.
- Serve the anti-inflammatory turmeric scrambled eggs with whole-grain toast or a side of mixed greens for a wholesome and satisfying breakfast.

NUTRITIONAL FACTS (PER SERVING):

- Calories: approximately 180 kcal
- Carbohydrates: 1g
- Protein: 12g
- Fat: 14g
- Fiber: 0g

Low-GI Avocado Toast with Poached Eggs

Prep Time:	Cook Time:	Serving Size:
10 minutes	5 minutes	2 persons

INGREDIENTS:

- 2 slices whole grain bread, toasted
- 1 ripe avocado, mashed
- 1 teaspoon fresh lemon juice
- Pepper and salt to taste
- 2 large eggs
- 1 teaspoon white vinegar
- Fresh arugula or spinach for topping

INSTRUCTIONS:

- In a bowl, combine the mashed avocado, fresh lemon juice, salt, and pepper. Blend the ingredients thoroughly until a smooth avocado paste is formed.
- Poach the eggs by filling a medium-sized saucepan with water, then add the white vinegar. Raise the heat to medium to bring the water to a gentle simmer.
- Open each egg into an individual cup or ramekin. With a spoon, gently stir the simmering water to create a whirlpool, and then cautiously lower each egg into the whirlpool's center, one by one. This will help the eggs stay compact and form a nice shape.
- Allow the eggs to poach in the water for roughly 3-4 minutes to achieve a soft, runny yolk, or extend the time if you prefer a harder yolk..
- While the eggs are poaching, spread the mashed avocado evenly on the toasted whole-grain bread slices.
- When the eggs have been poached to your liking, retrieve them from the water with a slotted spoon and position them atop the avocado-laden toast.
- Add a sprinkling of fresh arugula or spinach to each piece of toast, providing additional nutrients and a slight spiciness.
- Offer up the avocado toast crowned with poached eggs as a hearty and healthful choice for breakfast or brunch.

NUTRITIONAL FACTS (PER SERVING):

- Calories: approximately 250 kcal
- Carbohydrates: 19g
- Protein: 10g
- Fat: 16g
- Fiber: 8g

Metabolic-Boosting Green Smoothie Bowl

Prep Time:	**Cook Time:**	**Serving Size:**
5 minutes	0 minutes	2 persons

INGREDIENTS:

- 2 ripe bananas frozen
- 1 cup fresh spinach leaves
- 1 cup of non-sweetened almond milk (or any plant-based milk)
- 1 tablespoon chia seeds
- 1 tablespoon honey or maple syrup (optional for added sweetness)
- 1/2 avocado
- 1/2 cup chopped cucumber
- Fresh berries and sliced kiwi for topping
- Granola or nuts for added crunch (optional)

INSTRUCTIONS:

- In a blender, combine the fresh spinach leaves, frozen bananas, chopped cucumber, avocado, almond milk, chia seeds, and honey or maple syrup (if using).
- Blend the ingredients until smooth and creamy. The consistency can be tweaked by incorporating more almond milk if required.
- Divide the green smoothie into two bowls.
- Top each bowl with fresh berries, sliced kiwi, and granola or nuts (if using) for added texture and nutrients.
- Enjoy the metabolic-boosting green smoothie bowl as a refreshing and revitalizing breakfast or snack.

NUTRITIONAL FACTS (PER SERVING):

- Calories: approximately 300 kcal
- Carbohydrates: 45g
- Protein: 6g
- Fat: 13g
- Fiber: 10g

Almond Flour Pancakes with Berries

Prep Time:	Cook Time:	Serving Size:
10 minutes	10 minutes	2 persons

INGREDIENTS:

- 1 cup almond flour
- 2 large eggs
- 1/2 cup unsweetened almond milk (or any plant-based milk)
- 1 tablespoon honey or maple syrup
- 1/2 teaspoon baking powder
- 1/2 teaspoon pure vanilla extract
- Pinch of salt
- Fresh berries for topping
- Greek yogurt (optional)

INSTRUCTIONS:

- In a mixing bowl, whisk together the almond flour, eggs, almond milk, honey or maple syrup, baking powder, pure vanilla extract, and a pinch of salt until a smooth batter forms.
- Warm up a non-stick pan or griddle at medium heat, applying a small quantity of oil or cooking spray to prevent sticking.
- For each pancake, dispense approximately 1/4 cup of the pancake batter onto the heated surface.
- Allow the pancakes to cook for roughly 2-3 minutes on each side until they reach a golden brown color and are thoroughly cooked.
- Stack the almond flour pancakes on a plate and top them with fresh berries and a dollop of Greek yogurt if desired.
- Serve the almond flour pancakes with berries as a delicious and gluten-free breakfast treat.

NUTRITIONAL FACTS (PER SERVING):

- Calories: approximately 300 kcal
- Carbohydrates: 15g
- Protein: 13g
- Fat: 21g
- Fiber: 5g

Hormone-Balancing Chia Pudding

Prep Time:	Cook Time:	Serving Size:
10 minutes	0 minutes	2 persons

INGREDIENTS:

- 1/4 cup chia seeds
- 1 cup of non-sweetened almond milk (or any plant-based milk)
- 1 tablespoon chopped nuts (e.g., almonds, walnuts, or pistachios)
- 1 tablespoon pure maple syrup
- 1 tablespoon unsweetened shredded coconut
- 1/2 teaspoon pure vanilla extract
- 1/4 cup fresh berries (e.g., strawberries, blueberries, or raspberries)
- 1/4 teaspoon ground cinnamon

INSTRUCTIONS:

- Gather the chia seeds, almond milk, maple syrup, vanilla extract, and ground cinnamon in a mixing bowl. Stir thoroughly to make sure the chia seeds are uniformly dispersed.
- Allow the mixture to stand at room temperature for approximately 5 minutes, then give it another stir to prevent the seeds from clustering. After that, cover the bowl and place it in the refrigerator for at least 4 hours or overnight until the blend becomes thick and attains a pudding-like consistency.
- When it's time to dish up, split the chia pudding evenly into two bowls intended for serving.
- Enhance each serving with a topping of fresh berries, diced nuts, and grated coconut to introduce additional taste and texture.
- Enjoy the hormone-balancing chia pudding with your favorite herbal tea or as a light, nutritious dessert.

NUTRITIONAL FACTS (PER SERVING):

- Calories: approximately 220 kcal
- Carbohydrates: 24g
- Protein: 6g
- Fat: 12g
- Fiber: 11g

Veggie-Packed Breakfast Burritos

Prep Time:	Cook Time:	Serving Size:
15 minutes	15 minutes	2 persons

INGREDIENTS:

- 4 large eggs
- 1/4 cup diced bell peppers (assorted colors)
- 1/4 cup diced red onion
- 1/2 cup chopped spinach
- 1/2 cup diced tomatoes
- 1/4 cup shredded cheddar cheese
- 2 large whole wheat tortillas
- Pepper and salt to taste
- Cooking spray or a drizzle of olive oil

INSTRUCTIONS:

- Season the eggs with pepper and salt and whisk them in a bowl.
- Drizzle olive oil or apply a cooking spray lightly on a non-stick pan and warm it over medium heat.
- Incorporate the chopped red onion and bell peppers into the pan and sauté them for approximately 3 minutes until they start to lose their crispness.
- Integrate the chopped spinach and diced tomatoes into the mixture, allowing them to cook for an extra 2 minutes until the spinach has wilted.
- Gently pour the whisked eggs into the pan, mixing them softly with the vegetables. Keep cooking until the eggs are completely cooked and have a scrambled texture.
- Heat the whole wheat tortillas in a separate pan or briefly in the microwave until they become flexible.
- Distribute the mixture of scrambled eggs and vegetables evenly among the tortillas, placing it a bit off the center.
- Sprinkle the grated cheddar cheese over the top of the egg and vegetable blend.
- Fold the tortilla sides and roll it tightly to form a burrito-like shape.
- Slice the burritos in half and serve immediately as a delicious and nutrient-packed breakfast.

NUTRITIONAL FACTS (PER SERVING):

- Calories: approximately 340 kcal
- Carbohydrates: 25g
- Protein: 18g
- Fat: 17g
- Fiber: 5g

High-Protein Overnight Oats

Prep Time:	Cook Time:	Serving Size:
10 minutes	0 minutes	2 persons

INGREDIENTS:

- 1 cup rolled oats
- 1 1/2 cups almond milk, unsweetened (or any plant-based milk)
- 1/4 cup plain Greek yogurt
- 2 tablespoons chia seeds
- 1 tablespoon honey or maple syrup
- 1/2 teaspoon pure vanilla extract
- 1/4 cup sliced bananas
- 1/4 cup fresh berries (e.g., strawberries, blueberries, or raspberries)
- 2 tablespoons chopped nuts (e.g., almonds, walnuts, or pecans)

INSTRUCTIONS:

- Begin by blending the Greek yogurt, almond milk, chia seeds, rolled oats, and a splash of pure vanilla extract in a bowl. For a touch of sweetness, incorporate honey or maple syrup, stirring well until the mixture is homogenously combined.
- Divide the mixture into two jars or airtight containers, making sure there is enough room for expansion.
- Close the containers securely and store them in the fridge. They need to be kept for at least 4 hours, though leaving them overnight is ideal for the oats to soften as they soak up the liquid.
- Before you serve, make sure you stir the overnight oats well to combine all the elements.
- Top each portion with sliced bananas, fresh berries, and chopped nuts for added protein, flavor, and texture.
- Enjoy the high-protein overnight oats as a filling and wholesome breakfast to kickstart your day.

NUTRITIONAL FACTS (PER SERVING):

- Calories: approximately 350 kcal
- Carbohydrates: 45g
- Protein: 13g
- Fat: 13g
- Fiber: 10g

Spinach and Feta Frittata

Prep Time:	Cook Time:	Serving Size:
10 minutes	20 minutes	2 persons

INGREDIENTS:

- 4 large eggs
- 1/4 cup milk (any type)
- 1 cup fresh baby spinach leaves
- 1/4 cup crumbled feta cheese
- 1/4 cup diced red bell pepper
- 2 tablespoons diced red onion
- 1 tablespoon olive oil
- Pepper and salt to taste

INSTRUCTIONS:

- Get your oven warming up to 375°F (190°C).
- In a bowl, mix the milk, salt, eggs, and pepper together thoroughly using a whisk.
- Place an oven-safe skillet on medium heat and introduce the olive oil.
- For roughly 3-4 minutes, sauté the chopped red bell pepper and red onion in the skillet until they begin to become tender.
- Introduce the fresh baby spinach leaves to the skillet and allow them to cook for an extra 2 minutes until they have wilted.
- Spread the whisked egg mixture over the sautéed vegetables in the pan, ensuring uniform distribution.
- Scatter the crumbled feta cheese across the amalgamation of egg and vegetables.
- Allow the frittata to cook on the stovetop for roughly 3 minutes until you see the edges beginning to solidify.
- Shift the pan to a preheated oven and let it bake for an estimated 12-15 minutes until the frittata is thoroughly cooked and attains a light golden hue on top.
- Once done, take the skillet out of the oven, cut the frittata into slices, and serve it warm alongside a salad or a piece of rustic bread.

NUTRITIONAL FACTS (PER SERVING):

- Calories: approximately 260 kcal
- Carbohydrates: 7g
- Protein: 15g
- Fat: 19g
- Fiber: 2g

Nutty Granola with Greek Yogurt

Prep Time:	Cook Time:	Serving Size:
10 minutes	20 minutes	2 persons

INGREDIENTS:

- 1 cup rolled oats
- 1/4 cup chopped almonds
- 1/4 cup chopped walnuts
- 2 tablespoons honey
- 1 tablespoon coconut oil (melted)
- 1/2 teaspoon ground cinnamon
- Pinch of salt
- 1/4 cup dried cranberries or raisins
- 1 cup plain Greek yogurt

INSTRUCTIONS:

- Get your oven warming up to 325°F (165°C) and line a baking sheet with parchment paper.
- In a large mixing bowl, combine the chopped almonds, honey, melted coconut oil, chopped walnuts, ground cinnamon, rolled oats, and a pinch of salt. Blend vigorously so that everything is evenly covered.
- The granola mixture should be spread out evenly on the baking sheet.
- To make golden and crispy granola, bake in the heated oven for around 15-20 minutes, stirring once halfway through.
- Take the granola out of the oven and let it cool on the baking sheet.
- Add some dried fruit for sweetness once it's cooled down.
- To serve, divide the nutty granola into two portions and layer each portion with plain Greek yogurt in a bowl or glass.
- Combine the granola with a little Greek yogurt for a delicious and nutritious meal or snack.

NUTRITIONAL FACTS (PER SERVING):

- Calories: approximately 400 kcal
- Carbohydrates: 36g
- Protein: 20g
- Fat: 20g
- Fiber: 6g

Warming Cinnamon and Apple Porridge

Prep Time:	Cook Time:	Serving Size:
5 minutes	10 minutes	2 persons

INGREDIENTS:

- 1 cup rolled oats
- 2 cups unsweetened almond milk (or any plant-based milk)
- 1 apple, peeled, cored, and diced
- 1 tablespoon honey or maple syrup
- 1/2 teaspoon ground cinnamon
- Pinch of nutmeg
- Pinch of salt
- Chopped nuts and raisins for topping

INSTRUCTIONS:

- In a saucepan, combine the rolled oats, almond milk, diced apple, honey or maple syrup, ground cinnamon, nutmeg, and a pinch of salt.
- Over moderate temperatures, whisk the mixture regularly to keep it from sticking while it comes to a simmer.
- For oat tenderness and apple softness, cook the porridge for about 7 minutes.
- Divide the cinnamon and apple porridge into two serving bowls.
- Sprinkle some chopped nuts as well as raisins on top of each serving for a little of crunch and a touch of sweetness.
- Enjoy the warming cinnamon and apple porridge as a comforting and flavorful breakfast to start your day.

NUTRITIONAL FACTS (PER SERVING):

- Calories: approximately 300 kcal
- Carbohydrates: 50g
- Protein: 7g
- Fat: 8g
- Fiber: 8g

Black Bean Breakfast Quesadillas

Prep Time:	Cook Time:	Serving Size:
10 minutes	10 minutes	2 persons

INGREDIENTS:

- 4 small whole wheat tortillas
- 1 cup cooked black beans
- 1 cup diced bell peppers (assorted colors)
- 1/2 cup diced red onion
- 1 teaspoon ground cumin
- Pepper and salt to taste
- 1 cup shredded cheddar cheese (or any cheese of your choice)
- Salsa and sliced avocado for serving (optional)
- Cooking spray or a drizzle of olive oil
- 1/2 teaspoon chili powder

INSTRUCTIONS:

- In a bowl, mix the cooked black beans with diced bell peppers, red onion, ground cumin, chili powder, salt, and pepper.
- Warm up a non-stick frying pan over medium heat and lightly brush it with olive oil or cooking spray.
- Position one tortilla in the pan and uniformly spread half of the black bean mixture on its surface.

- Evenly scatter half of the grated cheddar cheese over the bean layer.
- Top with another tortilla to create a quesadilla, and press it gently with a spatula.
- Two to three minutes on every side should be enough time to toast the tortillas and melt the cheese in a quesadilla.
- To prepare another quesadilla, simply repeat the previous steps.
- If preferred, serve salsa and avocado slices alongside the quesadillas.

NUTRITIONAL FACTS (PER SERVING):

- Calories: approximately 400 kcal
- Carbohydrates: 45g
- Protein: 18g
- Fat: 15g
- Fiber: 10g

Spicy Scrambled Tofu

Prep Time:	Cook Time:	Serving Size:
10 minutes	10 minutes	2 persons

INGREDIENTS:

- 1 block of firm tofu, crumbled
- 2 tablespoons olive oil
- 1/2 cup diced tomatoes
- 1/4 cup chopped scallions (green onions)
- 1/4 cup chopped bell peppers (assorted colors)
- 2 cloves garlic, minced
- 1 teaspoon ground turmeric
- 1/2 teaspoon ground cumin
- 1/4 teaspoon cayenne pepper (adjust to taste)
- Pepper and salt to taste
- Fresh cilantro for garnish

INSTRUCTIONS:

- Put the olive oil in a big pan and heat it over medium heat.
- In a pan, over medium heat, add the crushed tofu and cook for 3 to 4 minutes, till it begins to brown.
- Stir in the diced tomatoes, chopped scallions, bell peppers, and minced garlic. To get desired tenderness in veggies, add 2 more minutes of cooking time.
- The tofu combination would benefit with the addition of ground cumin, cayenne pepper, salt, ground turmeric, and pepper. Mix well to evenly coat the tofu and vegetables with the spices.
- Continue cooking for another 2-3 minutes to let the flavors meld and the tofu absorb the spices.
- Remove the spicy scrambled tofu from the heat.
- For a blast of herbal freshness, dish the tofu scramble while it's still hot, topped with fresh cilantro.

NUTRITIONAL FACTS (PER SERVING):

- Calories: approximately 250 kcal
- Carbohydrates: 10g
- Protein: 15g
- Fat: 18g
- Fiber: 4g

Mushroom and Spinach Egg Muffins

Prep Time:	**Cook Time:**	**Serving Size:**
10 minutes	20 minutes	2 persons

INGREDIENTS:

- 4 large eggs
- 1 cup chopped mushrooms
- 1 cup chopped spinach
- 1/4 cup diced red bell pepper
- 1/4 cup diced red onion
- 1/2 cup shredded cheddar cheese (or any cheese of your choice)
- Pepper and salt to taste
- Cooking spray or a drizzle of olive oil

INSTRUCTIONS:

- Set your oven to preheat at 350°F (175°C) and prepare a muffin tin by lightly oiling it with cooking spray or olive oil.
- Take a bowl and whisk the eggs, seasoning them with a dash of pepper and salt.
- In a separate skillet, sauté the chopped mushrooms, spinach, red bell pepper, and red onion until the vegetables are tender.
- Divide the sautéed vegetables among the muffin cups in the tin.
- Fill each muffin tin approximately three-quarters of the way with the chopped veggies, then pour the beaten eggs on top.
- Top each muffin well with some shredded cheddar cheese.
- In a preheated oven, cook the egg muffins for 15 to 20 minutes, till the center is set and the top is lightly browned.
- Take the muffin tray out of the oven and wait a few minutes for the egg muffins to cool.

NUTRITIONAL FACTS (PER SERVING):

- Calories: approximately 200 kcal
- Carbohydrates: 6g
- Protein: 15g
- Fat: 13g
- Fiber: 2g

Buckwheat and Blueberry Breakfast Bowl

Prep Time:	Cook Time:	Serving Size:
5 minutes	15 minutes	2 persons

INGREDIENTS:

- 1 cup cooked buckwheat groats
- 1 cup of non-sweetened almond milk (or any plant-based milk)
- 1 tablespoon honey or maple syrup
- 1/2 teaspoon ground cinnamon
- Pinch of salt
- 1/2 cup fresh blueberries
- 1 tablespoon almond butter
- Chopped nuts and additional blueberries for topping

INSTRUCTIONS:

- In a saucepan, combine the cooked buckwheat groats, almond milk, honey or maple syrup, ground cinnamon, and a pinch of salt.
- Over medium heat, whisk the mixture regularly to prevent sticking and bring it to a boil.
- For a thicker or thinner porridge, cook the buckwheat for an additional few minutes.
- Divide the buckwheat and blueberry breakfast bowl into two serving bowls.
- Top each portion with fresh blueberries, a dollop of almond butter, and chopped nuts for added crunch and flavor.
- This wholesome and delicious buckwheat and blueberry breakfast dish is the perfect way to start your day.

NUTRITIONAL FACTS (PER SERVING):

- Calories: approximately 300 kcal
- Carbohydrates: 50g
- Protein: 8g
- Fat: 9g
- Fiber: 8g

CHAPTER 4

WHOLESOME LUNCHES

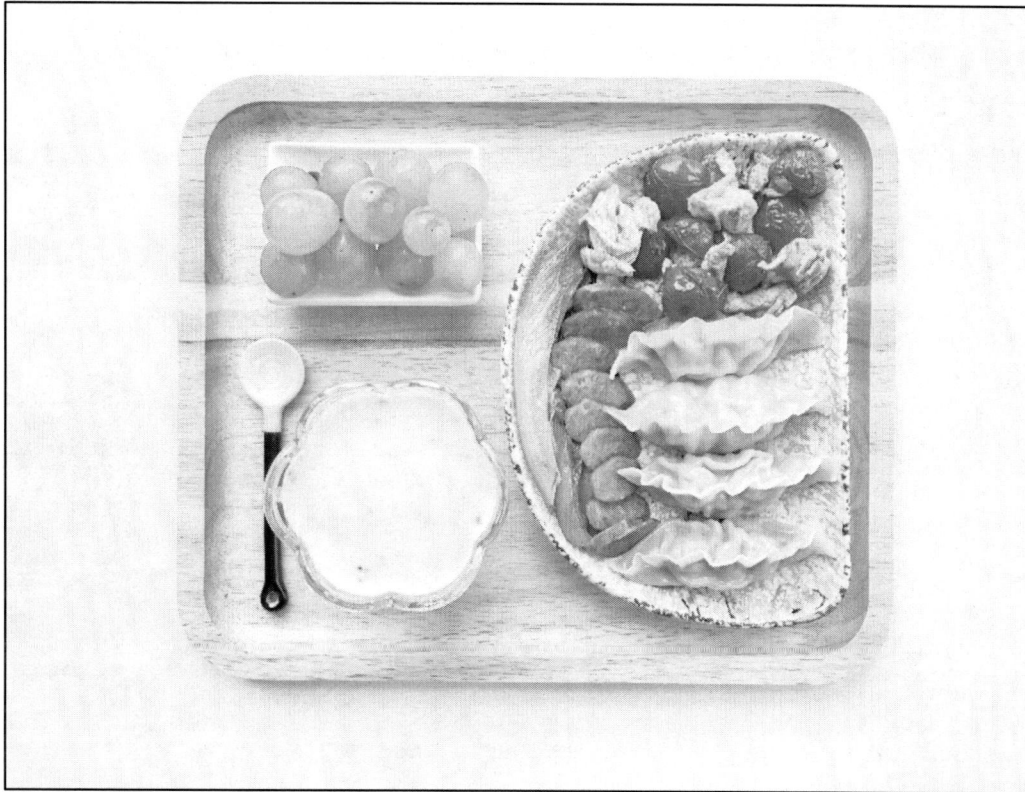

One of the key components in managing PCOS is a balanced and nutritious diet. Proper nutrition can help regulate hormone levels, manage weight, and improve overall health. In this chapter, we will explore 20 wholesome lunch recipes tailored specifically for PCOS patients. These recipes are not only delicious but also designed to promote hormonal balance and support the body's needs.

Nutritional Needs of PCOS Patients

Before we delve into the recipes, it is essential to understand the specific nutritional needs of PCOS patients. A well-balanced diet that focuses on complex carbohydrates, lean proteins, healthy fats, and fiber is crucial for managing PCOS symptoms effectively.

1. Nutrient-Dense Carbohydrates: Choose whole grains such as brown rice, oats, and quinoa over processed grains. These complex carbohydrates have a lower glycemic index, assisting in blood sugar regulation and avoiding insulin surges that could worsen PCOS symptoms.

2. Quality Proteins: Integrate protein sources like chicken, fish, turkey, legumes, and tofu into your diet. Proteins are critical for preserving muscle mass, fueling metabolism, and promoting satiety.

3. Beneficial Fats: Add healthy fats derived from avocados, nuts, seeds, and olive oil. These fats play a crucial role in hormone synthesis and the absorption of vitamins that are fat-soluble.

4. Fiber: Fiber-rich foods, including fruits, vegetables, and whole grains, are beneficial for digestion, prevention of insulin resistance, and weight control.

5. Foods Rich in Antioxidants: Consuming antioxidant-dense foods like various fruits and vegetables can decrease inflammation and oxidative stress within the body, which is helpful for individuals with PCOS.

20 RECIPES

Grilled Salmon Salad with Lemon Vinaigrette

Prep Time:	Cook Time:	Serving Size:
15 minutes	10 minutes	2 persons

INGREDIENTS:

- 2 salmon fillets
- 4 cups mixed salad greens (e.g., spinach, arugula, and lettuce)
- 1 cup cherry tomatoes, halved
- 1/2 cucumber, sliced
- 1/4 red onion, thinly sliced
- 1/4 cup crumbled feta cheese
- 2 tablespoons chopped fresh dill
- Pepper and salt to taste
- Lemon wedges for garnish

For the Lemon Vinaigrette:

- 3 tablespoons extra-virgin olive oil
- 1 tablespoon fresh lemon juice
- 1 teaspoon Dijon mustard
- 1 teaspoon honey
- Pepper and salt to taste

INSTRUCTIONS:

- Warm up your grill or a grilling pan to medium-high heat.
- Sprinkle the salmon fillets with a touch of pepper and salt for seasoning.
- Grill each side of the salmon fillets for approximately 4-5 minutes until they are fully cooked and mildly charred.
- Mix the mixed greens, cherry tomatoes, cucumber, red onion, crumbled feta cheese, and fresh dill in a spacious salad bowl.
- In a different, smaller bowl, stir together the components of the lemon vinaigrette until they blend well.
- Toss the salad with the lemon vinaigrette to coat the ingredients.
- Place the salmon fillets, which have been grilled, on top of the salad.
- Lemon slices make a great garnish.
- If you're looking for a light and filling meal, try the grilled salmon salad with lemon vinaigrette.

NUTRITIONAL FACTS (PER SERVING):

- Calories: approximately 400 kcal
- Carbohydrates: 12g
- Protein: 30g
- Fat: 26g
- Fiber: 3g

Quinoa-Stuffed Bell Peppers

Prep Time:	**Cook Time:**	**Serving Size:**
15 minutes	25 minutes	2 persons

INGREDIENTS:

- 2 large bell peppers (any color)
- 1 cup cooked quinoa
- 1 tablespoon olive oil
- 1 teaspoon ground cumin
- Pepper and salt to taste
- 1/2 cup cooked black beans
- 1/2 cup diced tomatoes
- 1/2 cup shredded cheddar cheese (or any cheese of your choice)
- 1/2 teaspoon chili powder
- 1/4 cup diced red onion
- 1/4 cup corn kernels (fresh, frozen, or canned)
- 1/4 cup chopped fresh cilantro

INSTRUCTIONS:

- Get your oven warming up to 375°F (190°C).
- Cut the tops off the bell peppers and remove the seeds and membranes from the inside.
- In a mixing bowl, combine the cooked quinoa, black beans, diced tomatoes, diced red onion, corn kernels, chopped fresh cilantro, olive oil, ground cumin, chili powder, salt, and pepper.
- Gently press the quinoa blend into the bell peppers, ensuring the filling is compact.
- Arrange the filled bell peppers on a baking tray and lightly cover them with aluminum foil.
- Allow the stuffed bell peppers to bake in the preheated oven for roughly 20 minutes.
- Take off the foil, spread the grated cheddar cheese over the stuffed peppers, and continue baking uncovered for another 5 minutes until the cheese is molten and bubbly.
- Serve the quinoa-stuffed bell peppers as a delicious and nutritious vegetarian meal.

NUTRITIONAL FACTS (PER SERVING):

- Calories: approximately 400 kcal
- Carbohydrates: 50g
- Protein: 15g
- Fat: 15g
- Fiber: 10g

Lentil and Sweet Potato Soup

Prep Time:	Cook Time:	Serving Size:
15 minutes	30 minutes	2 persons

INGREDIENTS:

- 1 cup dried red lentils, rinsed
- 1 large sweet potato, peeled and diced
- 1 carrot, peeled and diced
- 1 celery stalk, diced
- 1/2 onion, finely chopped
- 2 cloves garlic, minced
- 4 cups vegetable broth
- 1 teaspoon ground cumin
- 1/2 teaspoon ground coriander
- 1/4 teaspoon cayenne pepper (adjust to taste)
- Pepper and salt to taste
- 2 tablespoons chopped fresh parsley or cilantro for garnish

INSTRUCTIONS:

- In a large soup pot, sauté the chopped onion and minced garlic in a drizzle of olive oil over medium heat till they become fragrant and translucent.
- Add the diced sweet potato, carrot, and celery to the pot. Cook for a few minutes until the vegetables start to soften.
- Add the vegetable broth and add rinsed red lentils, ground cumin, ground coriander, cayenne pepper, salt, and pepper.
- Let the soup reach a boiling point, then lower the heat to maintain a gentle simmer for approximately 20-25 minutes until the lentils and vegetables achieve a soft texture.
- Use an immersion blender to partially blend the soup to your desired consistency. As another option, you could move a part of the soup to a blender, process it until it's smooth, and then pour it back into the pot.
- Adjust the seasoning if needed.
- Serve the lentil and sweet potato soup hot, garnished with chopped fresh parsley or cilantro.

NUTRITIONAL FACTS (PER SERVING):

- Calories: approximately 350 kcal
- Carbohydrates: 60g
- Protein: 15g
- Fat: 3g
- Fiber: 15g

Greek-Style Grilled Chicken Wraps

Prep Time:	Cook Time:	Serving Size:
15 minutes	15 minutes	2 persons

INGREDIENTS:

- 2 boneless, skinless chicken breasts
- 2 large whole wheat tortillas
- 1/2 cup plain Greek yogurt
- 1 tablespoon fresh lemon juice
- 1 clove garlic, minced
- 1 teaspoon dried oregano
- Pepper and salt to taste
- 1 cup shredded lettuce
- 1/2 cup diced cucumber
- 1/4 cup diced tomatoes
- 1/4 cup sliced Kalamata olives
- 1/4 cup crumbled feta cheese

INSTRUCTIONS:

- Warm up your grilling equipment, whether it's a grill or a grill pan, to a moderately high heat setting.
- Season the chicken breasts with pepper and salt.
- Grill the chicken for about 6-7 minutes per side till cooked through and nicely charred. Let it rest for a few minutes before slicing.
- In a small bowl, mix the plain Greek yogurt, fresh lemon juice, minced garlic, dried oregano, salt, and pepper to create a creamy Greek-style dressing.
- Lay the whole wheat tortillas flat on a clean surface.
- Spread a generous amount of Greek-style dressing on each tortilla.
- Arrange the shredded lettuce, diced cucumber, diced tomatoes, sliced Kalamata olives, and crumbled feta cheese on top of the dressing.
- Add the sliced grilled chicken to the center of each tortilla.
- Fold the sides of the tortillas over the filling and roll them up tightly to create the wraps.
- Serve the Greek-style grilled chicken wraps as a flavorful and satisfying lunch or dinner.

NUTRITIONAL FACTS (PER SERVING):

- Calories: approximately 450 kcal
- Carbohydrates: 35g
- Protein: 40g
- Fat: 18g
- Fiber: 7g

Spicy Chickpea Buddha Bowl

Prep Time:	**Cook Time:**	**Serving Size:**
15 minutes	10 minutes	2 persons

INGREDIENTS:

- 1 can (15 oz) chickpeas, drained and rinsed
- 1 tablespoon olive oil
- 1 teaspoon ground cumin
- 1/2 teaspoon smoked paprika
- 1/4 teaspoon cayenne pepper (adjust to taste)
- Pepper and salt to taste
- 2 cups cooked quinoa
- 1 cup shredded purple cabbage
- 1 cup sliced cucumber
- 1/2 cup grated carrots
- 1/2 avocado, sliced
- Fresh cilantro for garnish

For the Tahini Dressing:

- 3 tablespoons tahini
- 2 tablespoons fresh lemon juice
- 2 tablespoons water
- 1 clove garlic, minced
- Pepper and salt to taste

INSTRUCTIONS:

- In a large skillet, heat the olive oil over medium heat.
- Add the drained and rinsed chickpeas to the skillet.
- Sprinkle the ground cumin, smoked paprika, cayenne pepper, salt, and pepper over the chickpeas.
- Cook the chickpeas for about 5-7 minutes, stirring occasionally, until they are slightly crispy and well-coated with the spices.
- In a small bowl, whisk together the tahini, fresh lemon juice, water, minced garlic, salt, and pepper to create the tahini dressing.
- In two serving bowls, divide the cooked quinoa, shredded purple cabbage, sliced cucumber, grated carrots, and sliced avocado.
- Top each bowl with the spiced chickpeas.
- Drizzle the tahini dressing over the chickpea Buddha bowls.
- Garnish with fresh cilantro.
- Serve the spicy chickpea Buddha bowl as a nutrient-packed and flavorful plant-based meal.

NUTRITIONAL FACTS (PER SERVING):

- Calories: approximately 500 kcal
- Carbohydrates: 60g
- Protein: 20g
- Fat: 22g
- Fiber: 14g

Vegan Lentil Loaf with Tomato Glaze

Prep Time:	Cook Time:	Serving Size:
15 minutes	1 hour	2 persons

INGREDIENTS: FOR THE LENTIL LOAF:

- 1 cup cooked green lentils
- 1/2 cup rolled oats
- 1/2 cup finely chopped onions
- 1/2 cup grated carrots
- 1/2 cup bell peppers, chopped (any color)
- 2 cloves garlic, minced
- 1 tablespoon ground flaxseed mixed with 3 tablespoons water (flax egg)
- 2 tablespoons tomato paste
- 1 tablespoon soy sauce or tamari
- 1 teaspoon dried thyme
- 1 teaspoon dried oregano
- Pepper and salt to taste

For the Tomato Glaze:

- 1/4 cup tomato paste
- 2 tablespoons maple syrup or agave nectar
- 1 tablespoon apple cider vinegar
- 1/2 teaspoon smoked paprika
- 1/4 teaspoon garlic powder
- Pepper and salt to taste

INSTRUCTIONS:

- Get your oven warming up to 375°F (190°C) and lightly grease a loaf pan.

- In a large mixing bowl, combine the cooked lentils, rolled oats, chopped onions, grated carrots, chopped bell peppers, minced garlic, flax egg, tomato paste, soy sauce, dried thyme, dried oregano, salt, and pepper.
- Mix all the ingredients together until well combined.
- Transfer the lentil mixture to the loaf pan and spread it out evenly, pressing it down firmly.
- In a small bowl, whisk together the ingredients for the tomato glaze until smooth.
- Spread the tomato glaze evenly on top of the lentil loaf.
- Bake the lentil loaf in the preheated oven for about 45 minutes to 1 hour till it is firm and cooked through.
- Allow the lentil loaf to cool slightly before slicing and serving.

NUTRITIONAL FACTS (PER SERVING):

- Calories: approximately 350 kcal
- Carbohydrates: 65g
- Protein: 20g
- Fat: 4g
- Fiber: 15g

Turmeric-Spiced Cauliflower Stir-Fry

Prep Time:	Cook Time:	Serving Size:
10 minutes	15 minutes	2 persons

INGREDIENTS:

- 1 medium cauliflower, cut into florets
- 1 tablespoon olive oil
- 1 teaspoon ground turmeric
- 1/2 teaspoon ground cumin
- 1/4 teaspoon cayenne pepper (adjust to taste)
- Pepper and salt to taste
- 1 bell pepper, thinly sliced
- 1 cup sliced mushrooms
- 1 cup broccoli florets
- 2 cloves garlic, minced
- 2 tablespoons soy sauce or tamari
- 1 tablespoon sesame oil
- 2 green onions, sliced
- Sesame seeds for garnish

INSTRUCTIONS:

- In a large skillet or wok, heat the olive oil over medium heat.
- Add the cauliflower florets to the skillet and sprinkle with ground turmeric, ground cumin, cayenne pepper, salt, and pepper.
- Stir-fry the cauliflower for about 5 mins till it starts to become tender.
- Add the sliced bell pepper, sliced mushrooms, broccoli florets, and minced garlic to the skillet. Continue stir-frying for another 3-5 minutes until the vegetables are cooked to your desired level of crispness.
- Drizzle the soy sauce or tamari and sesame oil over the stir-fried vegetables. Toss to coat everything evenly.
- Garnish the turmeric-spiced cauliflower stir-fry with sliced green onions and sesame seeds.
- Serve the flavorful stir-fry as a delicious and nutritious vegan main or side dish.

NUTRITIONAL FACTS (PER SERVING):

- Calories: approximately 250 kcal
- Carbohydrates: 25g
- Protein: 10g
- Fat: 15g
- Fiber: 10g

Shrimp Avocado Salad with Citrus Dressing

Prep Time:	Cook Time:	Serving Size:
15 minutes	5 minutes	2 persons

INGREDIENTS:

- 1/2 pound cooked and peeled shrimp
- 1 ripe avocado, diced
- 1 cup cherry tomatoes, halved
- 1/4 cup diced red onion
- 1/4 cup chopped fresh cilantro
- 1 tablespoon olive oil
- 2 tablespoons fresh lemon juice
- 1 tablespoon fresh lime juice
- 1 teaspoon Dijon mustard
- Pepper and salt to taste
- Mixed greens for serving

INSTRUCTIONS:

- Blend the prepared shrimp, chopped avocado, sliced cherry tomatoes, diced red onion, and freshly cut cilantro in a big bowl.
- In a separate smaller bowl, mix together the olive oil, fresh lemon and lime juices, Dijon mustard, salt, and pepper to create a zesty citrus vinaigrette.
- Sprinkle the citrus vinaigrette over the shrimp and avocado combo, gently tossing to ensure all ingredients are covered with the dressing.
- Arrange a bed of mixed greens on serving plates or bowls.
- Spoon the shrimp avocado salad over the greens.
- Serve the refreshing shrimp avocado salad with citrus dressing as a light and satisfying lunch or dinner.

NUTRITIONAL FACTS (PER SERVING):

- Calories: approximately 300 kcal
- Carbohydrates: 14g
- Protein: 20g
- Fat: 20g
- Fiber: 7g

Mediterranean Farro Salad with Feta

Prep Time:	**Cook Time:**	**Serving Size:**
10 minutes	20 minutes	2 persons

INGREDIENTS:

- 1 cup cooked farro
- 1/2 cup diced cucumber
- 1/2 cup halved cherry tomatoes
- 1/4 cup diced red bell pepper
- 1/4 cup sliced Kalamata olives
- 2 tablespoons chopped fresh parsley
- 2 tablespoons crumbled feta cheese
- 1 tablespoon extra-virgin olive oil
- 1 tablespoon fresh lemon juice
- 1 clove garlic, minced
- Pepper and salt to taste

INSTRUCTIONS:

- In a large bowl, combine the cooked farro, diced cucumber, halved cherry tomatoes, diced red bell pepper, sliced Kalamata olives, chopped fresh parsley, and crumbled feta cheese.
- In a compact bowl, blend the minced garlic, fresh lemon juice, salt, pepper, and extra-virgin olive oil to prepare a lively dressing.
- Drizzle the dressing over the farro salad. Toss gently to coat all the ingredients with the dressing.
- Serve the Mediterranean farro salad with feta as a light and flavorful side dish or a satisfying lunch option.

NUTRITIONAL FACTS (PER SERVING):

- Calories: approximately 300 kcal
- Carbohydrates: 40g
- Protein: 10g
- Fat: 12g
- Fiber: 8g

Butternut Squash and Spinach Lasagna

Prep Time:	**Cook Time:**	**Serving Size:**
30 minutes	45 minutes	2 persons

INGREDIENTS:

- 6 lasagna noodles, cooked according to package instructions
- 2 cups butternut squash puree (cooked and mashed butternut squash)
- 1 cup chopped fresh spinach
- 1 cup ricotta cheese (or vegan ricotta substitute)
- 1 egg (or flax egg for a vegan option)
- 1 teaspoon dried oregano
- 1/2 cup shredded mozzarella cheese (or vegan mozzarella substitute)
- 1/2 teaspoon dried basil
- 1/4 cup grated Parmesan cheese (or vegan Parmesan substitute)
- 1/4 teaspoon ground nutmeg
- Pepper and salt to taste
- 1 cup marinara sauce

INSTRUCTIONS:

- Get your oven warming up to 375°F (190°C).
- In a mixing bowl, combine the butternut squash puree, chopped fresh spinach, ricotta cheese, shredded mozzarella cheese, grated Parmesan cheese, egg, dried oregano, dried basil, ground nutmeg, salt, and pepper.
- In a greased baking dish, layer the bottom with two cooked lasagna noodles.
- Spread half of the butternut squash and spinach mixture over the noodles.
- Add another layer of two lasagna noodles on top of the mixture.
- Spread the remaining butternut squash and spinach mixture over the noodles.
- Top with the final two lasagna noodles.
- Evenly distribute the marinara sauce over the uppermost layer of noodles.
- Cover the baking dish lightly with aluminum foil and allow it to bake in the preheated oven for 30 minutes.
- Remove the foil and sprinkle additional shredded mozzarella and grated Parmesan cheese on top.
- Bake uncovered for another 15 mins till the cheese is bubbly and golden.
- Let the butternut squash and spinach lasagna cool for a few minutes before slicing and serving.

NUTRITIONAL FACTS (PER SERVING):

- Calories: approximately 450 kcal
- Carbohydrates: 60g
- Protein: 20g
- Fat: 15g
- Fiber: 8g

Spiced Chicken and Veggie Skewers

Prep Time:	Cook Time:	Serving Size:
20 minutes	15 minutes	2 persons

INGREDIENTS:

- 2 boneless, skinless chicken breasts, cut into chunks
- 1 red bell pepper, cut into chunks
- 1 yellow bell pepper, cut into chunks
- 1 red onion, cut into chunks
- 1 zucchini, sliced into rounds
- 2 tablespoons olive oil
- 2 cloves garlic, minced
- 1 teaspoon ground cumin
- 1 teaspoon paprika
- 1/2 teaspoon chili powder
- Pepper and salt to taste
- Wooden or metal skewers

INSTRUCTIONS:

- Warm your grill or grilling pan to a medium-high temperature.
- Mix together the chunks of chicken, red and yellow bell peppers, red onion, and zucchini in a large bowl.
- In a different, smaller bowl, blend the olive oil, minced garlic, ground cumin, paprika, chili powder, salt, and pepper to concoct a spicy marinade.
- Pour the marinade over the chicken and veggie mixture. Toss to coat everything evenly.
- Thread the marinated chicken and veggies onto the skewers, alternating between different ingredients.
- Allow the skewers to grill for approximately 10-15 minutes, turning them intermittently, until the chicken is thoroughly cooked and the vegetables have a slight char.
- Serve the spiced chicken and veggie skewers as a delicious and colorful meal.

NUTRITIONAL FACTS (PER SERVING):

- Calories: approximately 350 kcal
- Carbohydrates: 15g
- Protein: 30g
- Fat: 20g
- Fiber: 5g

Black Bean and Corn Tacos

Prep Time:	**Cook Time:**	**Serving Size:**
15 minutes	10 minutes	2 persons

INGREDIENTS:

- 8 small corn tortillas
- 1 can (15 oz) black beans, drained and rinsed
- 1 cup diced tomatoes
- 1/4 cup diced red onion
- 1/4 cup chopped fresh cilantro
- 1 cup cooked corn kernels (fresh, frozen, or canned)
- 1 tablespoon olive oil
- 1 teaspoon ground cumin
- 1/2 teaspoon chili powder
- Pepper and salt to taste
- Sliced avocado and lime wedges for serving

INSTRUCTIONS:

- In a large skillet, heat the olive oil over medium heat.
- Add the drained and rinsed black beans, cooked corn kernels, diced tomatoes, diced red onion, chopped fresh cilantro, ground cumin, chili powder, salt, and pepper to the skillet.
- Cook the black bean and corn mixture for about 5-7 minutes, stirring occasionally, until heated through and well combined.
- Warm the corn tortillas in a separate dry skillet or microwave.
- Assemble the black bean and corn tacos by spooning the mixture onto each tortilla.
- Top with sliced avocado and squeeze fresh lime juice over the filling.
- Serve the tasty black bean and corn tacos as a satisfying and plant-based meal.

NUTRITIONAL FACTS (PER SERVING):

- Calories: approximately 350 kcal
- Carbohydrates: 55g
- Protein: 12g
- Fat: 10g
- Fiber: 12g

Zucchini Noodles with Avocado Pesto

Prep Time:	Cook Time:	Serving Size:
15 minutes	5 minutes	2 persons

INGREDIENTS:

- 2 large zucchini, spiralized into noodles
- 1 ripe avocado, pitted and peeled
- 1 cup fresh basil leaves
- 1/4 cup pine nuts or walnuts
- 2 tablespoons lemon juice
- 1 clove garlic, minced
- 2 tablespoons extra-virgin olive oil
- Pepper and salt to taste
- Cherry tomatoes and additional basil leaves for garnish

INSTRUCTIONS:

- In a blender or food processor, combine the ripe avocado, fresh basil leaves, pine nuts or walnuts, lemon juice, minced garlic, extra-virgin olive oil, salt, and pepper.
- Blend until the ingredients form a creamy and smooth avocado pesto sauce. If needed, add a splash of water to achieve the desired consistency.
- In a large skillet, lightly sauté the zucchini noodles over medium heat for about 2-3 minutes, just until they soften slightly. Avoid overcooking to maintain a bit of crunch.
- Toss the warm zucchini noodles with the avocado pesto sauce until well coated.
- Garnish with halved cherry tomatoes, and additional basil leaves for a pop of color and freshness.
- Serve the zucchini noodles with avocado pesto as a flavorful and nutritious gluten-free dish.

NUTRITIONAL FACTS (PER SERVING):

- Calories: approximately 400 kcal
- Carbohydrates: 20g
- Protein: 8g
- Fat: 35g
- Fiber: 10g

Warm Quinoa Salad with Roasted Veggies

Prep Time:	Cook Time:	Serving Size:
20 minutes	25 minutes	2 persons

INGREDIENTS:

- 1 cup cooked quinoa
- 1 cup diced sweet potatoes
- 1 cup diced zucchini
- 1 cup diced red bell pepper
- 1 tablespoon olive oil
- 1 teaspoon ground cumin
- 1/2 teaspoon paprika
- Pepper and salt to taste
- 2 cups baby spinach leaves
- 1/4 cup crumbled feta cheese (or vegan feta substitute)
- 2 tablespoons balsamic glaze (or balsamic vinegar reduction)

INSTRUCTIONS:

- Get your oven warming up to 400°F (200°C) and line a baking sheet with parchment paper.
- In a mixing bowl, toss the diced sweet potatoes, diced zucchini, and diced red bell pepper with olive oil, ground cumin, paprika, salt, and pepper until evenly coated.
- Spread the seasoned veggies in a single layer on the prepared baking sheet.
- Roast the vegetables in the preheated oven for about 20-25 minutes, stirring once halfway through, till they are tender and lightly caramelized.
- In a large bowl, combine the cooked quinoa, roasted veggies, and baby spinach leaves.
- Sprinkle the crumbled feta cheese over the quinoa and veggies.
- Drizzle the balsamic glaze or balsamic vinegar reduction on top for a burst of tangy sweetness.
- Toss the warm quinoa salad with roasted veggies until everything is well combined.
- Serve the hearty and colorful quinoa salad as a comforting and nourishing meal.

NUTRITIONAL FACTS (PER SERVING):

- Calories: approximately 400 kcal
- Carbohydrates: 50g
- Protein: 10g
- Fat: 18g
- Fiber: 10g

Grilled Eggplant Parmesan Stacks

Prep Time:	Cook Time:	Serving Size:
20 minutes	20 minutes	2 persons

INGREDIENTS:

- 1 large eggplant, cut into rounds
- 1 cup marinara sauce
- 1 cup shredded mozzarella cheese (or vegan mozzarella substitute)
- 1/4 cup grated Parmesan cheese (or vegan Parmesan substitute)
- 1/4 cup fresh basil leaves
- 2 tablespoons olive oil
- Pepper and salt to taste

INSTRUCTIONS:

- Warm up your grilling equipment, whether it's a grill or a grill pan, to a moderately high heat setting.
- Brush both sides of the eggplant rounds with olive oil and season with pepper and salt.
- Grill the eggplant rounds for about 2-3 minutes per side till they are tender and have grill marks.
- Get your oven warming up to 375°F (190°C).
- In a baking dish, layer the grilled eggplant rounds, spooning marinara sauce, shredded mozzarella cheese, and grated Parmesan cheese between each layer.
- Repeat the layers until all the eggplant is used, finishing with a layer of marinara sauce and cheese on top.
- Bake the eggplant Parmesan stacks in the preheated oven for about 15 mins till the cheese is melted and bubbly.
- Remove from the oven and garnish with fresh basil leaves.
- Serve the grilled eggplant Parmesan stacks as a delectable and comforting vegetarian dish.

NUTRITIONAL FACTS (PER SERVING):

- Calories: approximately 350 kcal
- Carbohydrates: 20g
- Protein: 15g
- Fat: 25g
- Fiber: 8g

Hearty Chicken and Vegetable Stew

Prep Time:	Cook Time:	Serving Size:
15 minutes	40 minutes	2 persons

INGREDIENTS:

- 2 boneless, skinless chicken breasts, cut into bite-sized pieces
- 1 tablespoon olive oil
- 1 onion, chopped
- 2 cloves garlic, minced
- 2 carrots, peeled and diced
- 2 celery stalks, diced
- 1 cup diced potatoes
- 1 cup diced tomatoes (canned or fresh)
- 4 cups chicken broth
- 1 teaspoon dried thyme
- 1 teaspoon dried rosemary
- Pepper and salt to taste
- 1 cup frozen peas
- Chopped fresh parsley for garnish

INSTRUCTIONS:

- In a large pot, heat the olive oil over medium heat.
- Introduce the finely chopped onion and minced garlic to the pot, sautéing until the onions attain a soft, translucent appearance.
- Add the cubed chicken into the pot and let it cook until it turns brown on all surfaces.
- Blend in the chopped carrots, celery, potatoes, and tomatoes.
- Incorporate the chicken broth into the mixture and season with dried thyme and rosemary.
- Add salt and pepper according to your preference.
- Elevate the stew to the boiling point, then diminish the heat to low, allowing it to simmer for around 30 minutes until the vegetables are adequately softened, and the flavors amalgamate.
- Mix in the frozen peas and allow them to cook for an extra 5 minutes until they're warmed through.
- Serve the robust chicken and vegetable stew in bowls and enhance it with a sprinkle of freshly chopped parsley.
- Serve the comforting stew as a satisfying and nourishing meal.

NUTRITIONAL FACTS (PER SERVING):

- Calories: approximately 400 kcal
- Carbohydrates: 40g
- Protein: 30g
- Fat: 12g
- Fiber: 8g

Tofu Pad Thai with Brown Rice Noodles

Prep Time:	Cook Time:	Serving Size:
20 minutes	15 minutes	2 persons

INGREDIENTS:

- 8 oz brown rice noodles
- 8 oz firm tofu, cubed
- 2 tablespoons vegetable oil
- 2 cloves garlic, minced
- 2 tablespoons tamarind paste
- 2 tablespoons soy sauce
- 1 tablespoon maple syrup or agave nectar
- 1 tablespoon rice vinegar
- 1 teaspoon chili garlic sauce (adjust to taste)
- 1 cup bean sprouts
- 1/2 cup chopped scallions
- 1/4 cup crushed peanuts
- Lime wedges for serving
- Fresh cilantro for garnish

INSTRUCTIONS:

- Prepare the brown rice noodles as per the instructions on the package. Once cooked, drain them and keep them aside.
- Heat the vegetable oil in a large frying pan or wok on medium-high heat.
- Sauté the tofu cubes in the skillet until they turn golden brown and crispy on all sides. Once done, remove and keep aside.
- In the same frying pan, add the minced garlic and sauté until it releases its aroma.
- In a separate bowl, blend tamarind paste, soy sauce, your choice of maple syrup or agave nectar, rice vinegar, and chili garlic sauce to create the Pad Thai sauce.
- Combine this sauce with the garlic in the skillet, stirring thoroughly.
- Introduce the cooked brown rice noodles to the skillet, ensuring they are evenly coated with the sauce by tossing them.
- Add the bean sprouts and chopped scallions to the skillet. Toss everything together until the vegetables are slightly wilted.
- Return the crispy tofu to the skillet and gently mix it into the Pad Thai.
- Divide the tofu Pad Thai with brown rice noodles into serving plates.
- Top each serving with crushed peanuts and garnish with fresh cilantro.
- Serve the delightful tofu Pad Thai as a flavorful and satisfying vegan meal.

NUTRITIONAL FACTS (PER SERVING):

- Calories: approximately 500 kcal
- Carbohydrates: 60g
- Protein: 18g
- Fat: 20g
- Fiber: 8g

Portobello Mushroom Burgers

Prep Time:	Cook Time:	Serving Size:
15 minutes	15 minutes	2 persons

INGREDIENTS:

- 2 large portobello mushroom caps
- 2 tablespoons balsamic vinegar
- 2 tablespoons olive oil
- 2 cloves garlic, minced
- 1 teaspoon dried thyme
- Pepper and salt to taste
- 4 whole wheat burger buns
- Baby spinach leaves for serving
- Sliced tomatoes for serving
- Sliced red onion for serving
- Avocado slices for serving

INSTRUCTIONS:

- In a shallow dish, whisk together the balsamic vinegar, olive oil, minced garlic, dried thyme, salt, and pepper.
- Place the portobello mushroom caps in the marinade, turning them to coat both sides. Let them marinate for about 10 minutes.
- Preheat your grill or grill pan over medium heat.
- Grill the marinated portobello mushroom caps for about 5-7 minutes per side till they are tender and slightly charred.
- Toast the burger buns on the grill for a minute till they are lightly golden.
- Assemble the Portobello mushroom burgers by placing baby spinach leaves on the bottom half of each burger bun.
- Add the grilled Portobello mushroom caps on top of the spinach.
- Top the mushrooms with sliced tomatoes, sliced red onion, and avocado slices.
- Place the top half of the burger bun on the stack to complete the burger.
- Serve the Portobello mushroom burgers as a delicious and wholesome vegetarian option.

NUTRITIONAL FACTS (PER SERVING):

- Calories: approximately 400 kcal
- Carbohydrates: 50g
- Protein: 10g
- Fat: 15g
- Fiber: 10g

Stuffed Acorn Squash with Wild Rice and Veggies

Prep Time:	Cook Time:	Serving Size:
20 minutes	40 minutes	2 persons

INGREDIENTS:

- 1 cup cooked wild rice
- 1 teaspoon dried thyme
- 1/2 cup diced bell peppers (any color)
- 1/2 cup diced eggplant
- 1/2 cup diced zucchini
- 1/2 teaspoon dried sage
- 1/4 cup chopped fresh parsley for garnish
- 1/4 cup diced red onion
- 2 cloves garlic, minced
- 2 small acorn squash, halved and seeds removed
- 2 tablespoons olive oil
- Pepper and salt to taste

INSTRUCTIONS:

- Get your oven warming up to 375°F (190°C).
- Place the halved acorn squash on a baking sheet, and cut side up.
- Spread olive oil over the halved acorn squash, then sprinkle dried thyme, dried sage, salt, and pepper for seasoning.
- Bake the acorn squash in the preheated oven for approximately 30 minutes or until they become tender and can be easily pierced with a fork.
- While the squash is being roasted, you can start preparing the stuffing. Warm a tablespoon of olive oil in a skillet over medium heat.
- Add the diced bell peppers, diced zucchini, diced eggplant, diced red onion, and minced garlic to the skillet.
- Sauté the vegetables until they are softened and slightly caramelized.
- Stir in the cooked wild rice and season with pepper and salt to taste.
- Once the acorn squash is done roasting, fill each squash half with the wild rice and vegetable stuffing.
- Garnish the stuffed acorn squash with chopped fresh parsley.
- Serve the delightful stuffed acorn squash with wild rice and veggies as a hearty and nutritious meal.

NUTRITIONAL FACTS (PER SERVING):

- Calories: approximately 400 kcal
- Carbohydrates: 60g
- Protein: 8g
- Fat: 15g
- Fiber: 12g

Grilled Tuna Salad with Avocado Salsa

Prep Time:	Cook Time:	Serving Size:
20 minutes	10 minutes	2 persons

INGREDIENTS:

- 2 tuna steaks
- 2 tablespoons olive oil
- 1 teaspoon smoked paprika
- Pepper and salt to taste
- 2 cups mixed salad greens
- 1 cup cherry tomatoes, halved
- 1/4 cup thinly sliced red onion
- 1/4 cup chopped cucumber
- 1 ripe avocado, diced
- 1 tablespoon lime juice
- 1 tablespoon chopped fresh cilantro
- 1 tablespoon chopped fresh mint
- 1 tablespoon chopped fresh parsley
- 1 tablespoon extra-virgin olive oil
- Pepper and salt to taste

INSTRUCTIONS:

- To begin, preheat the barbecue or grill pan on high heat.
- To prepare the tuna steaks, gently coat them with olive oil and then season them with smoked paprika, salt, along with pepper.
- To cook the tuna steaks, grill each side for approximately 2-3 minutes until they reach your preferred level of doneness. To maintain their juiciness, be cautious not to overcook them.
- Mixed salad greens, cherry tomato halves, red onion slices, and diced cucumber should be combined in a big bowl.
- To stop it from turning brown, combine the chopped avocado with the lime juice in a small bowl.
- Add the avocado, chopped fresh cilantro, chopped fresh mint, chopped fresh parsley, extra-virgin olive oil, salt, and pepper to the salad bowl.
- Toss everything together until the salad is well combined.
- Divide the grilled tuna salad with avocado salsa into serving plates.
- Serve the grilled tuna salad as a flavorful and nutritious dish.

NUTRITIONAL FACTS (PER SERVING):

- Calories: approximately 400 kcal
- Carbohydrates: 20g
- Protein: 35g
- Fat: 22g
- Fiber: 8g

CHAPTER 5

HEARTY DINNERS

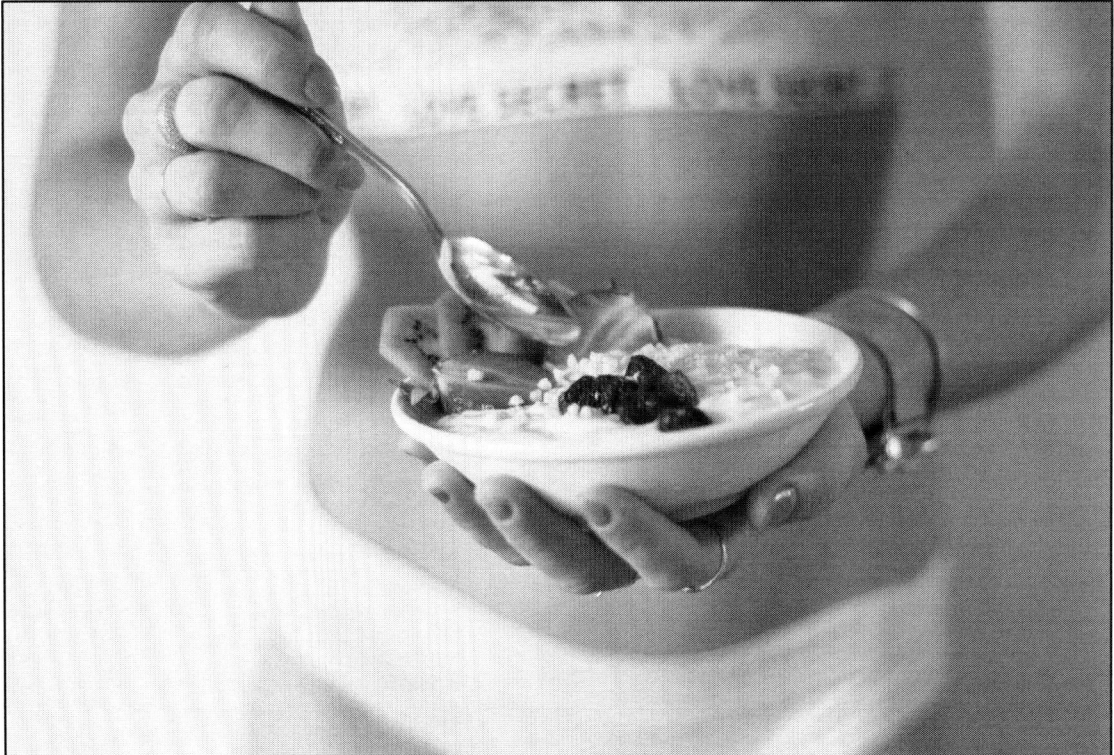

Polycystic Ovary Syndrome (PCOS) is a multifaceted hormonal disorder that affects the endocrine system and impacts millions of women around the world. Managing PCOS involves a holistic approach, and a crucial aspect of this is maintaining a balanced and nutritious diet. Dinner, being one of the main meals of the day, presents an excellent opportunity to provide the body with essential nutrients to support overall health and hormonal balance.

In this chapter, we have thoughtfully curated 20 delicious and nutrient-rich dinner recipes specially designed to cater to the needs of PCOS patients. Each recipe takes into account the dietary guidelines for managing PCOS, focusing on low glycemic index foods, anti-inflammatory ingredients, and a good balance of macronutrients. By incorporating these hearty dinners into their routine, PCOS patients can take proactive steps towards improved health and well-being.

20 RECIPES

Pan-Seared Salmon with Quinoa and Greens

Prep Time:	Cook Time:	Serving Size:
10 minutes	20 minutes	2 persons

INGREDIENTS:

- 2 salmon fillets
- 1 tablespoon olive oil
- Pepper and salt to taste
- 1 cup quinoa
- 2 cups vegetable broth or water
- 2 cups mixed greens (spinach, kale, arugula, etc.)
- 1 lemon, sliced for garnish

INSTRUCTIONS:

- Rinse the quinoa thoroughly under cold water.
- In a medium saucepan, bring the vegetable broth or water to a boil. Add the rinsed quinoa, reduce the heat to low, cover, and let it simmer for about 15-20 mins till the quinoa is cooked and the liquid is absorbed.
- While the quinoa is cooking, season the salmon fillets with pepper and salt.
- In a large skillet, heat the olive oil over medium-high heat.
- Place the salmon fillets into the skillet and cook for approximately 4-5 minutes on each side. This will ensure that the salmon is fully cooked and develops a golden crust.
- In the last few minutes of cooking the salmon, add the mixed greens to the skillet and sauté them until they wilt slightly.
- Divide the cooked quinoa and sautéed greens between two plates.
- Place a pan-seared salmon fillet on top of each bed of quinoa and greens.
- Garnish with lemon slices.
- Serve the pan-seared salmon with quinoa and greens as a healthy and flavorful meal.

NUTRITIONAL FACTS (PER SERVING):

- Calories: approximately 450 kcal
- Carbohydrates: 40g
- Protein: 35g
- Fat: 18g
- Fiber: 7g

Stuffed Chicken Breast with Spinach and Ricotta

Prep Time:	Cook Time:	Serving Size:
20 minutes	25 minutes	2 persons

INGREDIENTS:

- 2 boneless, skinless chicken breasts
- 1 cup chopped fresh spinach
- 1/2 cup ricotta cheese
- 2 tablespoons grated Parmesan cheese
- 1 clove garlic, minced
- 1 tablespoon olive oil
- Pepper and salt to taste
- Toothpicks or kitchen twine

INSTRUCTIONS:

- Get your oven warming up to 375°F (190°C).
- In a mixing bowl, combine the chopped fresh spinach, ricotta cheese, grated Parmesan cheese, minced garlic, olive oil, salt, and pepper.
- Slice a pocket horizontally into each chicken breast, being careful not to cut all the way through.
- Stuff each chicken breast with the spinach and ricotta mixture, and then secure the openings with toothpicks or tie them with kitchen twine to keep the stuffing intact.
- Put some olive oil in a pan that can go from the stovetop to the oven and heat it over medium heat.
- Sear the stuffed chicken breasts for about 2-3 minutes on each side until they are golden brown.
- Put the pan in the hot oven and bake for about 15-20 mins till the chicken is cooked through and no longer pink in the center.
- Remove the toothpicks or twine before serving.
- Serve the delicious stuffed chicken breast with spinach and ricotta as a hearty and satisfying dish.

NUTRITIONAL FACTS (PER SERVING):

- Calories: approximately 400 kcal
- Carbohydrates: 5g
- Protein: 40g
- Fat: 25g
- Fiber: 2g

Lentil and Vegetable Curry

Prep Time:	Cook Time:	Serving Size:
15 minutes	25 minutes	2 persons

INGREDIENTS:

- 1 cup dried lentils (red or green), rinsed and drained
- 2 tablespoons vegetable oil
- 1 onion, chopped
- 2 cloves garlic, minced
- 1 tablespoon grated ginger
- 1 tablespoon curry powder
- 1 teaspoon ground cumin
- 1 teaspoon ground coriander
- 1/2 teaspoon ground turmeric
- 1/4 teaspoon cayenne pepper (adjust to taste)
- 1 can (14 oz) diced tomatoes
- 1 cup vegetable broth or water
- 1 cup chopped vegetables (carrots, bell peppers, zucchini, etc.)
- 1 cup coconut milk
- Pepper and salt to taste
- Fresh cilantro for garnish
- Cooked rice for serving

INSTRUCTIONS:

- In a large pot or saucepan, heat the vegetable oil over medium heat.
- Add the chopped onion and sauté till it becomes translucent.
- Stir in the garlic and ginger that is grated, and cook for another minute until fragrant.
- Add the curry powder, ground cumin, ground coriander, ground turmeric, and cayenne pepper to the pot. Stir well to coat the onions and garlic with the spices.
- Pour in the diced tomatoes and vegetable broth or water, and bring the mixture to a simmer.
- Add the lentils and chopped vegetables to the pot. Cover and let the curry simmer for about 15-20 mins till the lentils are tender, and the vegetables are cooked.
- Stir in the coconut milk and let the curry simmer for an additional 5 minutes to meld the flavors together.
- Season the lentil and vegetable curry with pepper and salt to taste.
- Serve the flavorful lentil and vegetable curry over cooked rice, and garnish with fresh cilantro.

NUTRITIONAL FACTS (PER SERVING):

- Calories: approximately 400 kcal
- Carbohydrates: 50g
- Protein: 15g
- Fat: 15g
- Fiber: 15g

Sweet Potato and Black Bean Chili

Prep Time:	Cook Time:	Serving Size:
15 minutes	25 minutes	2 persons

INGREDIENTS:

- 1 tablespoon olive oil
- 1 onion, chopped
- 2 cloves garlic, minced
- 1 large sweet potato, peeled and diced
- 1 can (15 oz) black beans
- 1 can (14 oz) diced tomatoes
- 1 cup vegetable broth or water
- 2 tablespoons chili powder
- 1 teaspoon ground cumin
- 1/2 teaspoon smoked paprika
- 1/4 teaspoon cayenne pepper (adjust to taste)
- Pepper and salt to taste
- Fresh cilantro and sliced green onions
- Avocado slices for serving
- Cooked quinoa or rice for serving

INSTRUCTIONS:

- In a large pot or Dutch oven, heat the olive oil over medium heat.
- Add the chopped onion and sauté until it becomes translucent.
- Stir in the minced garlic and sauté for another minute until fragrant.
- Cook the diced sweet potato in the pot until it begins to soften for a few minutes.
- Combine black beans, diced tomatoes, and either vegetable broth or water in the pot.
- Add chili powder, ground cumin, smoked paprika, cayenne pepper, salt, and pepper, and stir thoroughly.
- Bring the mixture to a boil, then lower the heat, cover, and let it simmer for approximately 15-20 minutes until the sweet potatoes are tender and the flavors have blended perfectly.
- Serve the flavorful sweet potato and black bean chili over cooked quinoa or rice.
- Garnish with fresh cilantro, sliced green onions, and avocado slices.

NUTRITIONAL FACTS (PER SERVING):

- Calories: approximately 400 kcal
- Carbohydrates: 60g
- Protein: 15g
- Fat: 10g
- Fiber: 15g

Spaghetti Squash Pasta with Chunky Tomato Sauce

Prep Time:	Cook Time:	Serving Size:
15 minutes	45 minutes	2 persons

INGREDIENTS:

- 1 medium spaghetti squash
- 1 tablespoon olive oil
- 1 onion, chopped
- 2 cloves garlic, minced
- 1 can (14 oz) diced tomatoes
- 1 can (6 oz) tomato paste
- 1 teaspoon dried oregano
- 1 teaspoon dried basil
- 1/2 teaspoon dried thyme
- Pepper and salt to taste
- Grated Parmesan cheese (or vegan Parmesan substitute) for serving
- Fresh basil leaves for garnish

INSTRUCTIONS:

- Get your oven warming up to 375°F (190°C).
- Halve the spaghetti squash lengthwise and remove the seeds and stringy pulp.
- Coat the cut sides of the spaghetti squash with olive oil, then season with salt and pepper.
- Place the spaghetti squash halves cut-side down on a baking sheet lined with parchment paper.
- Roast the spaghetti squash in the preheated oven for about 35-40 mins till the flesh is tender and easily separates into spaghetti-like strands with a fork.
- While the squash is roasting, prepare the chunky tomato sauce. Using a saucepan, warm one tablespoon of olive oil on medium heat.
- Add the chopped onion and sauté until it becomes translucent.
- Stir in the minced garlic and sauté for another minute until fragrant.
- Add the diced tomatoes and tomato paste to the saucepan. Stir in the dried oregano, dried basil, dried thyme, salt, and pepper.
- Allow the tomato sauce to simmer for approximately 10-15 minutes, allowing the flavors to blend harmoniously.

- Once the spaghetti squash has finished roasting, use a fork to scrape the flesh, creating spaghetti-like strands.
- Divide the spaghetti squash pasta between two plates, and top with the chunky tomato sauce.
- Garnish with grated Parmesan cheese (or vegan Parmesan substitute) and fresh basil leaves.
- Serve the delightful spaghetti squash pasta with chunky tomato sauce as a nutritious and low-carb alternative to traditional pasta dishes.

NUTRITIONAL FACTS (PER SERVING):

- Calories: approximately 350 kcal
- Carbohydrates: 40g
- Protein: 10g
- Fat: 15g
- Fiber: 12g

Baked Cod with Zesty Lemon Sauce

Prep Time:	Cook Time:	Serving Size:
10 minutes	15 minutes	2 persons

INGREDIENTS:

- 2 cod fillets
- 2 tablespoons olive oil
- 2 tablespoons lemon juice
- 1 teaspoon lemon zest
- 2 cloves garlic, minced
- 1/2 teaspoon dried oregano
- Pepper and salt to taste
- Lemon slices and fresh parsley for garnish

INSTRUCTIONS:

- Get your oven warming up to 400°F (200°C).
- Prepare the zesty lemon sauce by whisking together olive oil, lemon juice, lemon zest, minced garlic, salt, dried oregano, and pepper in a small bowl.
- Take the cod fillets and arrange them in a baking dish. Pour the zesty lemon sauce over the fillets, ensuring they are thoroughly coated.
- Bake the cod in the preheated oven for approximately 12-15 minutes till the fish is fully cooked and reaches a point where it easily separates into flakes with a fork.
- Garnish with lemon slices and fresh parsley before serving.
- Serve the flavorful baked cod with zesty lemon sauce as a light and healthy seafood dish.

NUTRITIONAL FACTS (PER SERVING):

- Calories: approximately 300 kcal
- Carbohydrates: 1g
- Protein: 30g
- Fat: 20g
- Fiber: 0g

Vegan Shepherd's Pie

Prep Time:	Cook Time:	Serving Size:
20 minutes	35 minutes	2 persons

INGREDIENTS:

- 2 large potatoes, peeled and diced
- 2 tablespoons vegan butter or olive oil
- 1 onion, chopped
- 2 cloves garlic, minced
- 1 cup chopped carrots
- 1 cup chopped celery
- 1 cup chopped mushrooms
- 1 cup cooked lentils
- 1 cup vegetable broth
- 2 tablespoons tomato paste
- 1 teaspoon dried thyme
- Pepper and salt to taste
- 1 cup frozen peas
- Fresh parsley for garnish

INSTRUCTIONS:

- Cook the diced potatoes in a pot of salted water until they reach a tender consistency. Drain the potatoes and mash them using vegan butter or olive oil until a smooth texture is achieved. Set the mashed potatoes aside.

- On a large skillet, apply a small amount of oil and heat it over medium heat.
- Sauté the chopped onion and minced garlic until the onion turns translucent.
- Add the chopped carrots, chopped celery, and chopped mushrooms to the skillet. Cook until the vegetables are softened.
- Stir in the cooked lentils, vegetable broth, tomato paste, dried thyme, salt, and pepper. Let the mixture simmer for a few minutes until it thickens slightly.
- Get your oven warming up to 375°F (190°C).
- Move the lentil and vegetable mixture to a baking dish.
- Distribute the frozen peas over the lentil mixture.
- Evenly layer the mashed potatoes on top to cover the mixture.
- Bake the vegan shepherd's pie in the preheated oven for about 20 mins till the top is golden and slightly crispy.

- Garnish with fresh parsley before serving.
- Serve the hearty and comforting vegan shepherd's pie as a delicious plant-based meal.

NUTRITIONAL FACTS (PER SERVING):

- Calories: approximately 400 kcal
- Carbohydrates: 70g
- Protein: 15g
- Fat: 10g
- Fiber: 15g

Grilled Steak with Chimichurri Sauce

Prep Time:	**Cook Time:**	**Serving Size:**
15 minutes	10 minutes	2 persons

INGREDIENTS:

- 2 beef steak cuts (such as ribeye, sirloin, or flank)
- 2 tablespoons olive oil
- 2 cloves garlic, minced
- 1/4 cup chopped fresh parsley
- 2 tablespoons chopped fresh cilantro
- 1 tablespoon chopped fresh oregano
- 1/4 cup red wine vinegar
- 1/4 cup olive oil
- 1/4 teaspoon red pepper flakes (adjust to taste)
- Pepper and salt to taste
- Grilled vegetables for serving (optional)

INSTRUCTIONS:

- Begin by heating up your grill or grill pan at a high temperature.
- Season the steak cuts with olive oil, minced garlic, salt, and pepper, ensuring they are evenly coated.
- Grill the steaks for about 4-5 minutes per side till they reach your preferred level of doneness. Let them rest for a few minutes before slicing.
- Meanwhile, prepare the chimichurri sauce. In a bowl, combine the chopped fresh parsley, chopped fresh cilantro, chopped fresh oregano, olive oil, red pepper flakes, salt, red wine vinegar, and pepper. Mix well to create the sauce.
- Slice the grilled steaks and drizzle the chimichurri sauce over them.
- Serve the delicious grilled steak with chimichurri sauce as a mouthwatering and flavorful dish.
- You can also serve it with grilled vegetables for a complete and satisfying meal.

NUTRITIONAL FACTS (PER SERVING):

- Calories: approximately 500 kcal
- Carbohydrates: 2g
- Protein: 35g
- Fat: 40g
- Fiber: 1g

Oven-Baked Greek Chicken with Veggies

Prep Time:	Cook Time:	Serving Size:
15 minutes	30 minutes	2 persons

INGREDIENTS:

- 2 chicken breasts
- 2 tablespoons olive oil
- 2 cloves garlic, minced
- 1 teaspoon dried oregano
- 1/2 teaspoon dried thyme
- 1/2 teaspoon dried rosemary
- Juice of 1 lemon
- Pepper and salt to taste
- 1 cup cherry tomatoes, halved
- 1 cup sliced bell peppers (any color)
- 1 cup sliced zucchini
- 1/4 cup pitted Kalamata olives
- Fresh parsley for garnish

INSTRUCTIONS:

- Get your oven warming up to 400°F (200°C).
- In a bowl, mix together the minced garlic, salt, dried oregano, dried thyme, olive oil, dried rosemary, lemon juice, and pepper to make the marinade.
- Place the chicken breasts in a baking dish and pour the marinade over them, making sure they are well coated. Let them marinate for about 10-15 minutes.
- Add the halved cherry tomatoes, sliced bell peppers, sliced zucchini, and pitted Kalamata olives to the baking dish around the chicken.
- Bake the Greek chicken and veggies in the preheated oven for about 25-30 mins till the chicken is cooked through and the vegetables are tender.
- Garnish with fresh parsley before serving.
- Serve the flavorful oven-baked Greek chicken with veggies as a delightful and healthy Mediterranean-inspired dish.

NUTRITIONAL FACTS (PER SERVING):

- Calories: approximately 400 kcal
- Carbohydrates: 10g
- Protein: 30g
- Fat: 25g
- Fiber: 3g

Moroccan Chickpea Stew

Prep Time:	Cook Time:	Serving Size:
15 minutes	25 minutes	2 persons

INGREDIENTS:

- 1 tablespoon olive oil
- 1 onion, chopped
- 2 cloves garlic, minced
- 1 teaspoon ground cumin
- 1 teaspoon ground coriander
- 1/2 teaspoon ground turmeric
- 1/4 teaspoon ground cinnamon
- 1/4 teaspoon cayenne pepper (adjust to taste)
- Pepper and salt to taste
- 1 can (14 oz) diced tomatoes
- 2 cups cooked chickpeas (or 1 can, drained and rinsed)
- 2 cups vegetable broth
- 1 cup chopped sweet potatoes
- 1 cup chopped carrots
- 1 cup chopped bell peppers (any color)
- 1 cup chopped zucchini
- 1/4 cup chopped dried apricots (optional)
- Fresh cilantro for garnish
- Cooked couscous or rice for serving

INSTRUCTIONS:

- In a large pot or Dutch oven, heat the olive oil over medium heat.
- Add the chopped onion and sauté until it becomes translucent.
- Stir in the minced garlic, ground cumin, ground coriander, ground turmeric, ground cinnamon, cayenne pepper, salt, and pepper. Cook for another minute until the spices are fragrant.
- Pour in the diced tomatoes and vegetable broth. Stir in the cooked chickpeas, chopped sweet potatoes, chopped carrots, chopped bell peppers, chopped zucchini, and chopped dried apricots (if using).
- Let the stew simmer for about 15-20 mins till the vegetables are tender, and the flavors have melded together.
- Adjust the seasoning with more pepper and salt if needed.
- Serve the delightful Moroccan chickpea stew over cooked couscous or rice.

- Garnish with fresh cilantro before serving.
- Enjoy the flavorful and hearty Moroccan chickpea stew as a nourishing and exotic meal.

NUTRITIONAL FACTS (PER SERVING):

- Calories: approximately 400 kcal
- Carbohydrates: 60g
- Protein: 15g
- Fat: 10g
- Fiber: 15g

Shrimp and Veggie Stir-Fry with Brown Rice

Prep Time:	Cook Time:	Serving Size:
10 minutes	15 minutes	2 persons

INGREDIENTS:

- 1 cup cooked brown rice
- 8 oz shrimp, peeled and deveined
- 1 tablespoon vegetable oil
- 2 cloves garlic, minced
- 1 tablespoon grated ginger
- 1 cup broccoli florets
- 1 cup sliced bell peppers (any color)
- 1 cup sliced carrots
- 1 cup snap peas
- 2 tablespoons soy sauce
- 1 tablespoon oyster sauce (or vegetarian substitute)
- 1 teaspoon sesame oil
- 1 tablespoon sesame seeds for garnish
- Sliced green onions for garnish

INSTRUCTIONS:

- In a large skillet or wok, heat the vegetable oil over medium-high heat.
- Add the minced garlic and grated ginger to the skillet. Sauté for a minute until fragrant.
- Add the shrimp to the skillet and stir-fry until they turn pink and are cooked through. Remove the shrimp from the skillet and set them aside.
- In the same skillet, add a little more oil if needed, and sauté the broccoli, sliced bell peppers, sliced carrots, and snap peas until they are crisp-tender.
- Return the cooked shrimp to the skillet with the vegetables.
- In a small bowl, mix together the soy sauce, oyster sauce, and sesame oil. Pour the sauce over the shrimp and vegetables, and stir everything together until well coated.
- Serve the shrimp and veggie stir-fry over cooked brown rice.
- Garnish with sesame seeds and sliced green onions.
- Enjoy the delicious and nutritious shrimp and veggie stir-fry with brown rice.

NUTRITIONAL FACTS (PER SERVING):

- Calories: approximately 400 kcal
- Carbohydrates: 40g
- Protein: 30g
- Fat: 15g
- Fiber: 8g

Roasted Lemon Garlic Chicken with Veggies

Prep Time:	**Cook Time:**	**Serving Size:**
10 minutes	30 minutes	2 persons

INGREDIENTS:

- 2 boneless, skinless chicken breasts
- 2 tablespoons olive oil
- Juice of 1 lemon
- 2 cloves garlic, minced
- 1 teaspoon dried thyme
- 1 teaspoon dried rosemary
- Pepper and salt to taste
- 1 cup baby potatoes, halved
- 1 cup cherry tomatoes
- 1 cup green beans
- Lemon slices and fresh thyme for garnish

INSTRUCTIONS:

- Get your oven warming up to 400°F (200°C).
- In a bowl, whisk together the olive oil, lemon juice, minced garlic, dried thyme, dried rosemary, salt, and pepper to make the marinade.
- Place the chicken breasts in a baking dish and pour the marinade over them, ensuring they are well coated. Let them marinate for about 10 minutes.
- Add the halved baby potatoes, cherry tomatoes, and green beans to the baking dish around the chicken.
- Roast the lemon garlic chicken and veggies in the preheated oven for about 25-30 mins till the chicken is cooked through and the vegetables are tender.
- Garnish with lemon slices and fresh thyme before serving.
- Serve the succulent roasted lemon garlic chicken with veggies as a delightful and wholesome meal.

NUTRITIONAL FACTS (PER SERVING):

- Calories: approximately 450 kcal
- Carbohydrates: 25g
- Protein: 40g
- Fat: 20g
- Fiber: 6g

Turkey and Vegetable Meatloaf

Prep Time:	Cook Time:	Serving Size:
15 minutes	50 minutes	2 persons

INGREDIENTS:

- 1 lb ground turkey
- 1/2 cup breadcrumbs
- 1/4 cup grated Parmesan cheese
- 1/4 cup chopped fresh parsley
- 1/4 cup chopped onion
- 1/4 cup chopped bell peppers (any color)
- 1/4 cup shredded carrot
- 1/4 cup shredded zucchini
- 2 cloves garlic, minced
- 1 egg, lightly beaten
- 2 tablespoons ketchup
- 1 tablespoon Worcestershire sauce (or vegetarian substitute)
- 1 teaspoon dried oregano
- Pepper and salt to taste
- 1/4 cup ketchup for glaze

INSTRUCTIONS:

- Get your oven warming up to 375°F (190°C).
- In a large bowl, mix together the ground turkey, breadcrumbs, grated Parmesan cheese, chopped fresh parsley, chopped onion, chopped bell peppers, shredded carrot, shredded zucchini, minced garlic, lightly beaten egg, ketchup, Worcestershire sauce, dried oregano, salt, and pepper.
- Transfer the turkey and vegetable mixture to a loaf pan, shaping it into a loaf shape.
- Spread the ketchup evenly over the top of the meatloaf for the glaze.
- Bake the turkey and vegetable meatloaf in the preheated oven for about 45-50 mins till the internal temperature reaches 165°F (74°C).
- Let the meatloaf rest for a few minutes before slicing.
- Serve the delicious turkey and vegetable meatloaf with your favorite sides or vegetables.

NUTRITIONAL FACTS (PER SERVING):

- Calories: approximately 400 kcal
- Carbohydrates: 20g
- Protein: 30g
- Fat: 20g
- Fiber: 3g

Cauliflower Fried Rice with Tofu

Prep Time:	Cook Time:	Serving Size:
15 minutes	15 minutes	2 persons

INGREDIENTS:

- 1 small head of cauliflower, riced (about 2 cups)
- 8 oz firm tofu, cubed
- 2 tablespoons soy sauce
- 1 tablespoon sesame oil
- 1 tablespoon vegetable oil
- 1 cup chopped broccoli florets
- 1/2 cup shredded carrots
- 1/2 cup frozen peas
- 2 cloves garlic, minced
- 2 green onions, sliced
- Sesame seeds for garnish
- Sliced green onions for garnish

INSTRUCTIONS:

- To rice the cauliflower, chop the florets into small pieces and place them in a food processor. Pulse until they resemble rice-like grains.
- In a bowl, marinate the cubed tofu in soy sauce for a few minutes.
- In a large skillet or wok, heat the sesame oil and vegetable oil over medium-high heat.
- Add the marinated tofu to the skillet and stir-fry until it becomes golden and slightly crispy. Remove the tofu from the skillet and set it aside.
- In the same skillet, sauté the chopped broccoli florets, shredded carrots, and frozen peas until they are tender-crisp.
- Add the minced garlic and sliced green onions to the skillet. Cook for another minute until fragrant.
- Stir in the riced cauliflower and cook for a few minutes until it becomes tender.
- Return the cooked tofu to the skillet with the cauliflower and vegetables.
- Drizzle with additional soy sauce if desired, and mix everything together until well combined.
- Serve the delicious cauliflower fried rice with tofu.
- Garnish with sesame seeds and sliced green onions before serving.
- Enjoy the flavorful and healthy cauliflower fried rice as a satisfying and nutritious alternative to traditional fried rice.

NUTRITIONAL FACTS (PER SERVING):

- Calories: approximately 350 kcal
- Carbohydrates: 20g
- Protein: 20g
- Fat: 20g
- Fiber: 8g

Oven-Baked Salmon with Lemon Dill Sauce

Prep Time:	Cook Time:	Serving Size:
10 minutes	15 minutes	2 persons

INGREDIENTS:

- 2 salmon fillets
- 2 tablespoons olive oil
- Juice of 1 lemon
- 2 cloves garlic, minced
- 1 teaspoon dried dill
- Pepper and salt to taste
- Lemon slices for garnish
- Fresh dill for garnish

INSTRUCTIONS:

- Get your oven warming up to 400°F (200°C).
- In a small bowl, whisk together the olive oil, lemon juice, minced garlic, dried dill, salt, and pepper to make the marinade.
- Place the salmon fillets in a baking dish and pour the marinade over them, making sure they are well coated.
- Bake the salmon in the preheated oven for about 12-15 mins till the fish is cooked through and flakes easily with a fork.
- Garnish with lemon slices and fresh dill before serving.
- Serve the oven-baked salmon with lemon dill sauce as a delightful and nutritious seafood dish.

NUTRITIONAL FACTS (PER SERVING):

- Calories: approximately 400 kcal
- Carbohydrates: 1g
- Protein: 30g
- Fat: 30g
- Fiber: 0g

Ratatouille with Quinoa

Prep Time:	Cook Time:	Serving Size:
15 minutes	30 minutes	2 persons

INGREDIENTS:

- 1 cup quinoa
- 2 cups vegetable broth or water
- 2 tablespoons olive oil
- 1 onion, chopped
- 2 cloves garlic, minced
- 1 eggplant, diced
- 1 zucchini, diced
- 1 yellow squash, diced
- 1 red bell pepper, diced
- 1 can (14 oz) diced tomatoes
- 1 teaspoon dried thyme
- 1 teaspoon dried oregano
- Pepper and salt to taste
- Fresh basil leaves for garnish

INSTRUCTIONS:

- Rinse the quinoa thoroughly under cold water.
- In a medium saucepan, bring the vegetable broth or water to a boil. Add the rinsed quinoa, reduce the heat to low, cover, and let it simmer for about 15-20 mins till the quinoa is cooked and the liquid is absorbed.
- In a large skillet, heat the olive oil over medium heat.
- Add the chopped onion and sauté until it becomes translucent.
- Stir in the minced garlic and sauté for another minute until fragrant.
- Add the diced eggplant, diced zucchini, diced yellow squash, and diced red bell pepper to the skillet. Cook until the vegetables are tender.
- Pour in the diced tomatoes, dried thyme, dried oregano, salt, and pepper. Stir everything together and let the ratatouille simmer for a few minutes to meld the flavors.
- Serve the ratatouille over cooked quinoa.
- Garnish with fresh basil leaves before serving.
- Enjoy the flavorful ratatouille with quinoa as a delightful and healthy vegetable-packed dish.

NUTRITIONAL FACTS (PER SERVING):

- Calories: approximately 400 kcal
- Carbohydrates: 60g
- Protein: 10g
- Fat: 15g
- Fiber: 10g

Lemon Herb Roasted Chicken with Brussels Sprouts

Prep Time:	**Cook Time:**	**Serving Size:**
10 minutes	25 minutes	2 persons

INGREDIENTS:

- 2 boneless, skinless chicken breasts
- 2 tablespoons olive oil
- Juice of 1 lemon
- 2 cloves garlic, minced
- 1 teaspoon dried thyme
- 1 teaspoon dried rosemary
- Pepper and salt to taste
- 1 lb Brussels sprouts, trimmed and halved
- Lemon slices for garnish
- Fresh parsley for garnish

INSTRUCTIONS:

- Get your oven warming up to 400°F (200°C).
- In a bowl, whisk together the olive oil, lemon juice, minced garlic, dried thyme, dried rosemary, salt, and pepper to make the marinade.
- Place the chicken breasts and halved Brussels sprouts in a baking dish.
- Pour the marinade over the chicken and Brussels sprouts, making sure they are well coated.
- Bake the lemon herb roasted chicken and Brussels sprouts in the preheated oven for about 20-25 mins till the chicken is cooked through and the Brussels sprouts are tender and slightly crispy.
- Garnish with lemon slices and fresh parsley before serving.
- Serve the succulent lemon herb roasted chicken with Brussels sprouts as a flavorful and nutritious meal.

NUTRITIONAL FACTS (PER SERVING):

- Calories: approximately 450 kcal
- Carbohydrates: 20g
- Protein: 40g
- Fat: 20g
- Fiber: 8g

Stuffed Bell Peppers with Ground Turkey and Veggies

Prep Time:	Cook Time:	Serving Size:
20 minutes	35 minutes	2 persons

INGREDIENTS:

- 2 large bell peppers (any color)
- 1 tablespoon olive oil
- 1/2 lb ground turkey
- 1/2 cup chopped onion
- 1/2 cup chopped mushrooms
- 1/2 cup chopped zucchini
- 1 clove garlic, minced
- 1 teaspoon dried oregano
- 1 teaspoon dried basil
- Pepper and salt to taste
- 1 cup cooked quinoa (from Recipe 1)
- 1/2 cup shredded mozzarella cheese (optional)
- Fresh parsley for garnish

INSTRUCTIONS:

- Get your oven warming up to 375°F (190°C).
- Cut the tops off the bell peppers and remove the seeds and membranes from the inside. Set the bell peppers aside.
- In a large skillet, heat the olive oil over medium heat.
- Add the ground turkey to the skillet and cook until it is browned and cooked through. Break the turkey into crumbles while cooking.
- Stir in the chopped onion, chopped mushrooms, chopped zucchini, and minced garlic. Cook until the vegetables are tender.
- Season the mixture with dried oregano, dried basil, salt, and pepper.
- Stir in the cooked quinoa and shredded mozzarella cheese (if using) into the turkey and vegetable mixture until well combined.
- Stuff the bell peppers with the turkey and quinoa mixture, pressing it down gently.
- Place the stuffed bell peppers in a baking dish.

- Bake the stuffed bell peppers in the preheated oven for about 25-30 mins till the peppers are tender.
- Garnish with fresh parsley before serving.
- Serve the delicious stuffed bell peppers with ground turkey and veggies as a satisfying and wholesome meal.

NUTRITIONAL FACTS (PER SERVING):

- Calories: approximately 450 kcal
- Carbohydrates: 30g
- Protein: 30g
- Fat: 20g
- Fiber: 8g

Spinach and Mushroom Risotto

Prep Time:	Cook Time:	Serving Size:
10 minutes	25 minutes	2 persons

INGREDIENTS:

- 1 cup Arborio rice
- 4 cups vegetable broth or chicken broth
- 2 tablespoons butter
- 1 tablespoon olive oil
- 1/2 cup chopped onion
- 2 cloves garlic, minced
- 1 cup sliced mushrooms
- 2 cups fresh spinach leaves
- 1/4 cup grated Parmesan cheese
- Pepper and salt to taste
- Fresh parsley for garnish

INSTRUCTIONS:

- In a medium saucepan, heat the vegetable broth or chicken broth over low heat to keep it warm.
- In a large skillet or saucepan, heat the butter and olive oil over medium heat.
- Add the chopped onion and sauté until it becomes translucent.
- Stir in the minced garlic and sauté for another minute until fragrant.
- Add the Arborio rice to the skillet and cook for a few minutes until it becomes lightly toasted.
- Gradually add the warm vegetable broth or chicken broth, about one ladleful at a time, stirring constantly and allowing the liquid to be absorbed before adding more.
- Continue this process until the risotto becomes creamy and the rice is tender but still has a slight bite (about 20-25 minutes).
- In the last few minutes of cooking, stir in the sliced mushrooms and fresh spinach leaves. Cook until the mushrooms are tender and the spinach wilts.
- Stir in the grated Parmesan cheese and season with pepper and salt to taste.
- Serve the creamy spinach and mushroom risotto as a comforting and flavorful dish.
- Garnish with fresh parsley before serving.

NUTRITIONAL FACTS (PER SERVING):

- Calories: approximately 400 kcal
- Carbohydrates: 60g
- Protein: 10g
- Fat: 15g
- Fiber: 5g

Baked Tilapia with Zucchini Noodles

Prep Time:	Cook Time:	Serving Size:
15 minutes	15 minutes	2 persons

INGREDIENTS:

- 2 tilapia fillets
- 2 tablespoons olive oil
- Juice of 1 lemon
- 2 cloves garlic, minced
- 1 teaspoon dried thyme
- 1 teaspoon paprika
- Pepper and salt to taste
- 2 zucchinis, spiralized into noodles
- Lemon wedges and fresh dill for garnish

INSTRUCTIONS:

- Get your oven warming up to 400°F (200°C).
- In a bowl, whisk together the olive oil, lemon juice, minced garlic, dried thyme, paprika, salt, and pepper to make the marinade.
- Place the tilapia fillets in a baking dish and pour the marinade over them, making sure they are well coated.
- Bake the tilapia in the preheated oven for about 10-15 mins till the fish is cooked through and flakes easily with a fork.
- In a separate skillet, heat a little olive oil over medium heat.
- Add the zucchini noodles and sauté for a few minutes until they are tender-crisp.
- Serve the baked tilapia over the sautéed zucchini noodles.
- Garnish with lemon wedges and fresh dill before serving.
- Enjoy the light and flavorful baked tilapia with zucchini noodles as a healthy and satisfying seafood dish.

NUTRITIONAL FACTS (PER SERVING):

- Calories: approximately 350 kcal
- Carbohydrates: 10g
- Protein: 30g
- Fat: 20g
- Fiber: 3g

CHAPTER 6

SATISFYING SNACKS

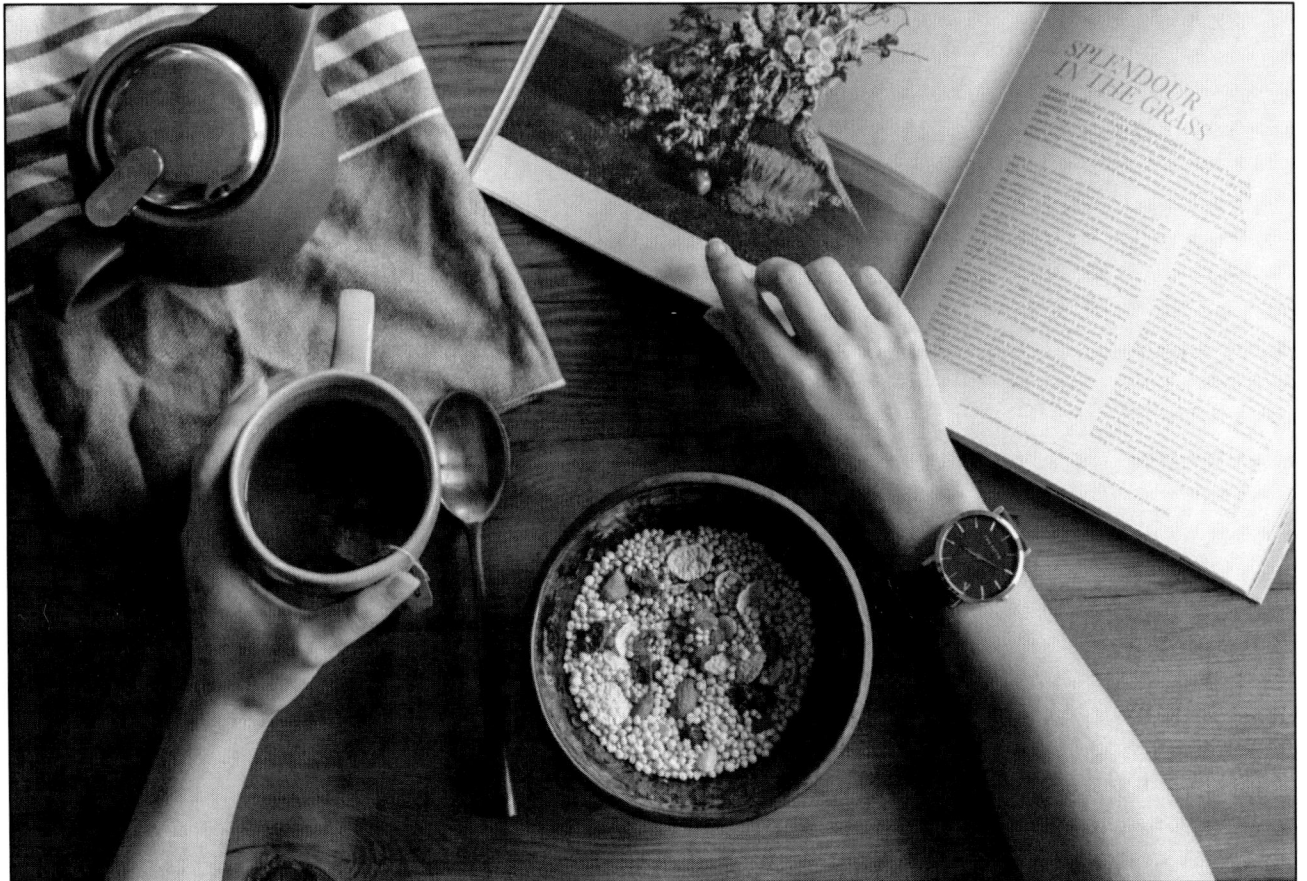

If you've been diagnosed with PCOS, you're probably wondering what you should consume for meals and snacks. If you're like many of the women we work with, you've probably already read a lot about eating for PCOS on the internet or through podcasts. Due to information overload and all of the conflicting advice available, you may even feel MORE confused as you research. This post will break things down for you and provide you with options for PCOS-friendly foods.

Things to Consider When Making PCOS Snacks

70% of PCOS cases are caused by insulin resistance. Elevated insulin and blood sugar levels cause food cravings, making it harder to make healthy meal choices. Your body craves sugar, and it craves it right now! Addressing this component with the appropriate lifestyle modifications is critical, and our functional medicine program assists women in doing so. Women with adrenal and inflammatory PCOS should continue to monitor their blood sugar levels. When our bodies are in "fight or flight" mode, high cortisol levels can contribute to elevated blood sugar. When we think of "snacks," we often think of items with poor nutritional density, such as chips and pretzels. We aim to change this perspective and think of snacks as "mini meals" that help address dietary gaps by providing extra fiber, healthy fats, protein, and phytonutrients (from colorful fruits and vegetables).

Do I Need to Eat Something?

Before reaching for a snack, consider the following:

Is it really that you're hungry, or are you eating out of habit? Consider a hunger scale ranging from 0 to 10, with 0 being voracious hunger and 10 being so full you need to unbutton your pants. To avoid cravings and overeating, strive to keep your hunger rating between 3 and 7 throughout the day. It will take some trial and error to figure out what food combinations work best for you (hint: it will be difficult to stay in this range without the right macronutrient balance). Is it because you didn't eat enough protein and fat at breakfast or lunch that you're hungry? Eating pure carbohydrates (for example, a breakfast of plain oats, fruit, and orange juice) guarantees hunger and food desires throughout the day. Experiment with various food combinations and keep track of how satiated you feel afterward.

Should Certain Women Abstain from Snacking?

You are the expert on your own body and the only one who knows what it requires. Some women with severe insulin resistance may benefit from eating three balanced meals per day with no snacks in between, as this allows their insulin levels to be lower throughout the day. Getting to the point where you only eat three meals per day with no snacks can be difficult and time-consuming (for the reasons described above, as well as the food cravings that accompany insulin-resistant PCOS). To successfully avoid snacking while you have PCOS, meticulous preparation and the addition of healthy fats, proteins, and brightly colored plant foods at each meal are required. In our Foundational Meal Plan, we provide ideas for balanced meals. The idea is not for you to consume a low-calorie diet and feel hungry all day. Snacks to avoid Eating enough calories, fat, vitamins, and minerals is actually necessary for optimal hormone production.

Avoid eating basic "naked" carbohydrates as snacks. Plain crackers, chips, popcorn, and pretzels, for example, are low in protein, fat, and fiber. These snacks will not fill you up, so you will be more likely to overeat or seek out another snack an hour later. You may also be tempted to eat basic fruits or vegetables as a snack since it appears to be the "healthy" thing to do, but eating produce alone is unlikely to be a fulfilling snack in the absence of protein and fat.

The Best PCOS Snacks

The ideal snacks for PCOS will tick several boxes Fiber (complex carbs), Protein Fat that is good for you. Include a brightly colored fruit or vegetable, as well as Omega-3 fatty acids (such as walnuts, flax, chia, or sardines). They are filling enough to keep you going for 2–4 hours.

In this comprehensive chapter, we will delve into 15 delicious and nutritious snack recipes tailored specifically for PCOS patients. These snacks are designed to be satisfying, easy to prepare, and packed with essential nutrients that can significantly benefit those with PCOS. From savory to sweet options, there's something for everyone to enjoy while adhering to a PCOS-friendly diet.

15 RECIPES

Almond Butter Energy Balls

Prep Time:	**Chill Time:**	**Serving Size:**
15 minutes	30 minutes	Makes about 12 energy balls

INGREDIENTS:

- 1 cup rolled oats
- 1/2 cup almond butter
- 1/4 cup honey or maple syrup
- 1/4 cup ground flaxseed
- 1/4 cup shredded coconut (unsweetened)
- 1 teaspoon vanilla extract
- Pinch of salt
- Optional add-ins: chocolate chips, chopped nuts, dried fruits

INSTRUCTIONS:

- In a large mixing bowl, combine rolled oats, almond butter, honey or maple syrup, ground flaxseed, shredded coconut, vanilla extract, and a pinch of salt.
- If desired, add in some chocolate chips, chopped nuts, or dried fruits to enhance the flavor and texture.
- Stir all the ingredients together until well combined.
- Refrigerate the mixture for about 20-30 minutes to make it easier to handle.
- Once chilled, take a tablespoon of the mixture and roll it between your palms to form a compact ball. Repeat with the remaining mixture.
- Place the almond butter energy balls on a plate or baking sheet lined with parchment paper.
- Chill the energy balls in the refrigerator for an additional 10-15 minutes to set.
- Once they are firm, transfer the energy balls to an airtight container and store them in the refrigerator for up to a week.
- Enjoy these nutritious and delicious almond butter energy balls as a quick and energizing snack.

Nutritional facts (per energy ball):

- Calories: approximately 100 kcal
- Carbohydrates: 10g
- Protein: 3g
- Fat: 6g
- Fiber: 2g

Baked Sweet Potato Chips

Prep Time:	**Bake Time:**	**Serving Size:**
10 minutes	20-25 minutes	Serves 2-3 persons

INGREDIENTS:

- 2 medium sweet potatoes, washed and peeled
- 2 tablespoons olive oil
- 1 teaspoon paprika
- 1/2 teaspoon garlic powder
- 1/2 teaspoon onion powder
- Pepper and salt to taste

INSTRUCTIONS:

- Get your oven warming up to 375°F (190°C).
- Thinly slice the peeled sweet potatoes using a mandoline slicer or a sharp knife. Aim for uniform thickness to ensure even baking.
- In a large bowl, toss the sweet potato slices with olive oil, paprika, garlic powder, onion powder, salt, and pepper. Make sure the slices are evenly coated with the seasoning.
- Arrange the seasoned sweet potato slices in a single layer on a baking sheet lined with parchment paper.
- Bake the sweet potato chips in the preheated oven for about 20-25 mins till they become crispy and slightly golden. Check them occasionally to prevent burning.
- Once baked, remove the sweet potato chips from the oven and let them cool slightly before serving.
- Enjoy the wholesome and crunchy baked sweet potato chips as a healthier alternative to store-bought chips.

NUTRITIONAL FACTS (PER SERVING):

- Calories: approximately 150 kcal
- Carbohydrates: 20g
- Protein: 2g
- Fat: 7g
- Fiber: 4g

Spiced Roasted Chickpeas

Prep Time:	Bake Time:	Serving Size:
10 minutes	25-30 minutes	Serves 2-3 persons

INGREDIENTS:

- 1 can (14 oz) chickpeas (garbanzo beans), drained and rinsed
- 1 tablespoon olive oil
- 1 teaspoon ground cumin
- 1/2 teaspoon smoked paprika
- 1/4 teaspoon cayenne pepper (adjust to taste)
- Pepper and salt to taste

INSTRUCTIONS:

- Get your oven warming up to 400°F (200°C).
- Pat the chickpeas dry with a paper towel to remove excess moisture.
- In a bowl, toss the chickpeas with olive oil, ground cumin, smoked paprika, cayenne pepper, salt, and pepper. Make sure the chickpeas are evenly coated with the spices.
- Spread the spiced chickpeas in a single layer on a baking sheet lined with parchment paper.
- Bake the chickpeas in the preheated oven for about 25-30 mins till they become crispy and golden brown. Shake the pan or stir the chickpeas halfway through baking for even roasting.
- Once roasted, remove the chickpeas from the oven and let them cool slightly before serving.
- Enjoy the flavorful and crunchy spiced roasted chickpeas as a protein-packed and satisfying snack.

NUTRITIONAL FACTS (PER SERVING):

- Calories: approximately 130 kcal
- Carbohydrates: 15g
- Protein: 6g
- Fat: 5g
- Fiber: 5g

Apple Slices with Almond Butter

Prep Time:

5 minutes

Serving Size:

Serves 2 persons

INGREDIENTS:

- 2 apples (your favorite variety), cored and sliced
- 4 tablespoons almond butter
- Optional toppings: honey, cinnamon, chopped nuts, dried fruits

NUTRITIONAL FACTS (PER SERVING):

- Calories: approximately 200 kcal
- Carbohydrates: 30g
- Protein: 4g
- Fat: 9g
- Fiber: 6g

INSTRUCTIONS:

- Wash and core the apples, then slice them into thin rounds or sticks.
- Arrange the apple slices on a plate or serving tray.
- Place the almond butter in a small dipping bowl.
- Serve the apple slices with almond butter for dipping.
- If desired, drizzle a little honey over the almond butter or sprinkle some cinnamon on top. You can also add chopped nuts or dried fruits for extra flavor and texture.
- Enjoy the simple and nutritious apple slices with almond butter as a delicious and satisfying snack.

Hummus with Veggie Sticks

Prep Time:	**Serving Size:**
10 minutes	Serves 2-3 persons

INGREDIENTS:

- 1 cup canned chickpeas (garbanzo beans), drained and rinsed
- 1/4 cup tahini (sesame paste)
- 2 cloves garlic, minced
- 2 tablespoons lemon juice
- 2 tablespoons olive oil
- 2-4 tablespoons water
- Pepper and salt to taste
- Assorted veggie sticks (carrots, cucumber, bell peppers, celery, etc.) for dipping

INSTRUCTIONS:

- In a food processor or blender, combine the canned chickpeas, tahini, minced garlic, lemon juice, olive oil, and a pinch of pepper and salt.
- Blend the ingredients until smooth and creamy. If the hummus is too thick, add water a tablespoon at a time and continue blending until desired consistency is achieved.
- Taste the hummus and adjust the seasoning with more pepper and salt if needed.
- Transfer the hummus to a serving bowl.
- Wash and cut assorted veggies into sticks for dipping.
- Arrange the veggie sticks around the hummus bowl for serving.
- Enjoy the creamy and flavorful hummus with veggie sticks as a healthy and delightful snack or appetizer.

NUTRITIONAL FACTS (PER SERVING):

- Calories: approximately 150 kcal
- Carbohydrates: 10g
- Protein: 5g
- Fat: 10g
- Fiber: 4g

Baked Zucchini Fries

Prep Time:	**Bake Time:**	**Serving Size:**
15 minutes	20-25 minutes	Serves 2-3 persons

INGREDIENTS:

- 2 medium zucchinis, washed and cut into fry-like shapes
- 1/2 cup panko breadcrumbs (or regular breadcrumbs)
- 1/4 cup grated Parmesan cheese
- 1 teaspoon garlic powder
- 1 teaspoon dried oregano
- 1/2 teaspoon paprika
- Pepper and salt to taste
- 2 large eggs, beaten
- Cooking spray or olive oil

INSTRUCTIONS:

- Get your oven warming up to 425°F (220°C). Line a baking sheet with parchment paper or aluminum foil and lightly grease it with cooking spray or olive oil.
- In a shallow dish, mix the panko breadcrumbs, grated Parmesan cheese, garlic powder, dried oregano, paprika, salt, and pepper.
- Dip the zucchini sticks into the beaten eggs, allowing any excess to drip off.
- Roll the egg-coated zucchini sticks in the breadcrumb mixture, pressing the breadcrumbs onto the zucchini to adhere.
- Place the coated zucchini fries on the prepared baking sheet in a single layer.
- Lightly spray the zucchini fries with cooking spray or drizzle them with olive oil to help them become crispy during baking.
- Bake the zucchini fries in the preheated oven for about 20-25 mins till they are golden and crispy.
- Serve the baked zucchini fries with your favorite dipping sauce or ketchup for a healthier twist on a classic snack.

NUTRITIONAL FACTS (PER SERVING):

- Calories: approximately 150 kcal
- Carbohydrates: 15g
- Protein: 8g
- Fat: 7g
- Fiber: 3g

Greek Yogurt with Honey and Berries

Prep Time:

5 minutes

Serving Size:

Serves 2 persons

INGREDIENTS:

- 1 cup Greek yogurt
- 2 tablespoons honey
- Assorted fresh berries (strawberries, blueberries, raspberries)
- Optional toppings: granola, chopped nuts, mint leaves

NUTRITIONAL FACTS (PER SERVING):

- Calories: approximately 200 kcal
- Carbohydrates: 25g
- Protein: 12g
- Fat: 6g
- Fiber: 2g

INSTRUCTIONS:

- In a serving bowl, spoon the Greek yogurt.
- Drizzle the honey over the yogurt, adjusting the amount to your desired sweetness.
- Top the yogurt with a generous amount of assorted fresh berries.
- If desired, sprinkle some granola or chopped nuts over the yogurt for added crunch and flavor.
- Garnish with fresh mint leaves for a touch of freshness.
- Enjoy the creamy and tangy Greek yogurt with honey and berries as a delightful and refreshing snack or breakfast.

Spicy Tuna Stuffed Avocados

Prep Time:	**Serving Size:**
10 minutes	Serves 2 persons

INGREDIENTS:

- 2 ripe avocados, halved and pitted
- 1 can (5 oz) tuna, drained
- 2 tablespoons mayonnaise
- 1 tablespoon Sriracha sauce (adjust to taste)
- 1 tablespoon lime juice
- Pepper and salt to taste
- Optional toppings: chopped cilantro, sliced jalapeños

INSTRUCTIONS:

- In a bowl, flake the drained tuna with a fork.
- Stir in the mayonnaise, Sriracha sauce, lime juice, salt, and pepper until well combined.
- Adjust the amount of Sriracha sauce to your preferred level of spiciness.
- Spoon the spicy tuna mixture into the halved and pitted avocados, dividing it equally among the halves.
- If desired, sprinkle chopped cilantro or add sliced jalapeños on top for extra flavor and heat.
- Serve the spicy tuna stuffed avocados as a satisfying and nutritious snack or light meal.

NUTRITIONAL FACTS (PER SERVING):

- Calories: approximately 300 kcal
- Carbohydrates: 10g
- Protein: 15g
- Fat: 25g
- Fiber: 8g

Trail Mix with Nuts and Dark Chocolate

Prep Time:

5 minutes

Serving Size:

Serves 2 persons

INGREDIENTS:

- 1/2 cup almonds
- 1/2 cup cashews
- 1/2 cup peanuts
- 1/4 cup dark chocolate chips or chunks
- 1/4 cup dried cranberries or raisins
- 1/4 cup dried apricots, chopped

INSTRUCTIONS:

- In a mixing bowl, combine the almonds, cashews, peanuts, dark chocolate chips or chunks, dried cranberries or raisins, and chopped dried apricots.
- Toss the ingredients together until they are well mixed.
- Transfer the trail mix to a resealable bag or an airtight container for storage.
- Enjoy the delicious and satisfying trail mix as a portable and energy-boosting snack for on-the-go moments or outdoor activities.

NUTRITIONAL FACTS (PER SERVING):

- Calories: approximately 350 kcal
- Carbohydrates: 20g
- Protein: 10g
- Fat: 25g
- Fiber: 5g

Pumpkin Seeds with Sea Salt

Prep Time:	Roast Time:	Serving Size:
5 minutes	10-15 minutes	Serves 2 persons

INGREDIENTS:

- 1 cup raw pumpkin seeds (pepitas)
- 1 tablespoon olive oil
- Sea salt to taste

INSTRUCTIONS:

- Get your oven warming up to 350°F (175°C).
- In a bowl, toss the raw pumpkin seeds with olive oil until they are evenly coated.
- Spread the pumpkin seeds in a single layer on a baking sheet lined with parchment paper or aluminum foil.
- Sprinkle sea salt over the pumpkin seeds to your desired level of saltiness.
- Roast the pumpkin seeds in the preheated oven for about 10-15 mins till they become lightly golden and crispy.
- Remove the roasted pumpkin seeds from the oven and let them cool before serving.
- Enjoy nutritious and crunchy pumpkin seeds with sea salt as a delightful and healthy snack.

NUTRITIONAL FACTS (PER SERVING):

- Calories: approximately 200 kcal
- Carbohydrates: 4g
- Protein: 10g
- Fat: 15g
- Fiber: 2g

Ants on a Log (Celery with Peanut Butter and Raisins)

Prep Time:
5 minutes

Serving Size:
Serves 2 persons

INGREDIENTS:

- 4 celery stalks, washed and trimmed
- 2 tablespoons peanut butter (or any nut or seed butter of your choice)
- 2 tablespoons raisins

INSTRUCTIONS:

- Cut each celery stalk into smaller sticks, approximately 3-4 inches in length.
- Spread peanut butter along the center of each celery stick.
- Press raisins into the peanut butter, creating an "ants on a log" effect.
- Arrange the filled celery sticks on a plate or serving platter.
- Enjoy the fun and nutritious ants on a log as a delightful snack or appetizer.

NUTRITIONAL FACTS (PER SERVING):

- Calories: approximately 150 kcal
- Carbohydrates: 15g
- Protein: 4g
- Fat: 8g
- Fiber: 3g

Greek Salad Skewers

Prep Time:

15 minutes

Serving Size:

Makes about 6 skewers

INGREDIENTS:

- 1 cup cherry tomatoes
- 1 cup cucumber, cut into bite-sized pieces
- 1 cup feta cheese, cut into cubes
- 1/2 cup Kalamata olives
- 2 tablespoons extra-virgin olive oil
- 1 tablespoon red wine vinegar
- 1 teaspoon dried oregano
- Pepper and salt to taste
- Wooden skewers

INSTRUCTIONS:

- Thread cherry tomatoes, cucumber pieces, feta cheese cubes, and Kalamata olives onto the wooden skewers in any desired order.
- In a small bowl, whisk together extra-virgin olive oil, red wine vinegar, dried oregano, salt, and pepper to make the dressing.
- Drizzle the dressing over the Greek salad skewers just before serving.

- Serve the colorful and flavorful Greek salad skewers as a refreshing and healthy appetizer or party snack.

NUTRITIONAL FACTS (PER SKEWER):

- Calories: approximately 100 kcal
- Carbohydrates: 5g
- Protein: 5g
- Fat: 7g
- Fiber: 1g

Guacamole with Cucumber Slices

Prep Time:	Serving Size:
10 minutes	Serves 2 persons

INGREDIENTS:

- 2 ripe avocados, peeled and pitted
- 1/4 cup finely chopped onion
- 1 small tomato, diced
- 1 jalapeño (seeds removed for milder flavor), finely chopped
- 1 clove garlic, minced
- Juice of 1 lime
- Pepper and salt to taste
- Cucumber slices for serving

INSTRUCTIONS:

- In a bowl, mash the peeled and pitted avocados with a fork until smooth.
- Stir in the finely chopped onion, diced tomato, finely chopped jalapeño, minced garlic, and lime juice.
- Season the guacamole with pepper and salt to taste. Adjust the amount of lime juice and jalapeño for the preferred taste and spiciness.
- Transfer the guacamole to a serving bowl.
- Serve the delicious and creamy guacamole with cucumber slices for dipping or spreading.

NUTRITIONAL FACTS (PER SERVING):

- Calories: approximately 250 kcal
- Carbohydrates: 15g
- Protein: 4g
- Fat: 20g
- Fiber: 10g

Oven-Baked Kale Chips

Prep Time:	**Bake Time:**	**Serving Size:**
10 minutes	10-15 minutes	Serves 2 persons

INGREDIENTS:

- 1 bunch of fresh kale, washed and dried
- 1 tablespoon olive oil
- 1/2 teaspoon garlic powder
- 1/2 teaspoon paprika
- Salt to taste

INSTRUCTIONS:

- Get your oven warming up to 350°F (175°C).
- Remove the tough stems from the kale leaves and tear the leaves into bite-sized pieces.
- In a large mixing bowl, toss the kale pieces with olive oil until they are evenly coated.
- Sprinkle garlic powder, paprika, and salt over the kale, tossing again to distribute the seasonings.
- Spread the seasoned kale pieces in a single layer on a baking sheet lined with parchment paper.
- Bake the kale chips in the preheated oven for about 10-15 mins till they become crispy and slightly golden.
- Keep an eye on the kale chips while baking to avoid burning.
- Once baked, remove the kale chips from the oven and let them cool slightly before serving.
- Enjoy the crispy and nutritious oven-baked kale chips as a guilt-free and flavorful snack.

NUTRITIONAL FACTS (PER SERVING):

- Calories: approximately 100 kcal
- Carbohydrates: 7g
- Protein: 3g
- Fat: 7g
- Fiber: 3g

Caprese Salad Bites

Prep Time:	**Serving Size:**
10 minutes	Makes about 12 bites

INGREDIENTS:

- 12 cherry tomatoes
- 12 small fresh mozzarella balls (bocconcini)
- Fresh basil leaves
- Balsamic glaze or balsamic reduction (store-bought or homemade)

INSTRUCTIONS:

- ◆ Wash the cherry tomatoes and pat them dry.
- ◆ Thread a cherry tomato, a small fresh mozzarella ball, and a fresh basil leaf onto a toothpick or small skewer.
- ◆ Repeat the process until you have assembled all the Caprese salad bites.
- ◆ Arrange the Caprese salad bites on a serving platter or plate.
- ◆ Drizzle balsamic glaze or balsamic reduction over the Caprese bites just before serving.

- ◆ Serve these delightful and elegant Caprese salad bites as a tasty and appetizing party snack or appetizer.

Nutritional facts (per bite):

- Calories: approximately 50 kcal
- Carbohydrates: 1g
- Protein: 3g
- Fat: 4g
- Fiber: 0g

CHAPTER 7

DELECTABLE DESSERTS

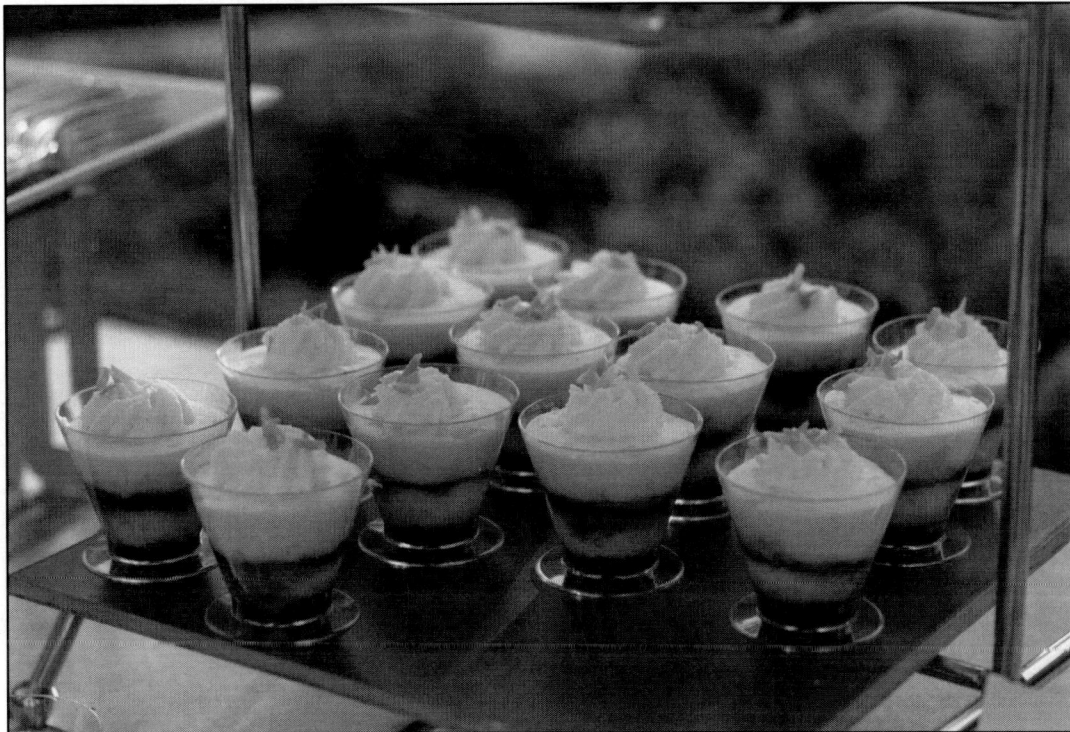

I n the world of culinary delights, few things evoke as much joy and satisfaction as desserts. These sweet indulgences have a magical ability to put a smile on anyone's face, turning an ordinary meal into a memorable feast. From classic favorites to innovative creations, the realm of desserts offers an endless array of options to please every palate. In this chapter, we will explore fifteen exquisite dessert recipes, each crafted to perfection, promising to tantalize your taste buds and leave you craving for more.

Following a PCOS diet does not imply deprivation. Not even remotely. If you have PCOS, you can indulge in a variety of delectable sweet delights. All it takes is replacing standard items with PCOS-friendly alternatives. These healthy options taste just as wonderful as their conventional counterparts, and the majority of them are insanely simple to prepare.

So, how do you make a healthy yet luscious PCOS dessert? Let us investigate.

WHAT IS A PCOS-FRIENDLY DESSERT?

A PCOS-friendly dessert contains fewer carbohydrates, dairy products, and added sugars. Most recipes use alternative flour instead of all-purpose flour, and many use milk replacements such as almond or oat milk instead of dairy milk. These dairy-free vanilla cupcakes are also low in carbs. Let's talk about what you should and shouldn't use in a PCOS dessert.

Ingredients to stay away from

Most PCOS-friendly dessert recipes minimize or exclude common baking ingredients such as milk, sugar, and all-purpose flour.

Milk: According to Verywell Health, carbs like milk might raise insulin and testosterone levels. If you have PCOS, experts recommend decreasing your dairy consumption.

According to the Open-Heart Journal, sugar can cause an increase in insulin levels. In one animal study, rats developed PCOS after eating a high-fat, high-sugar diet. PCOS Nutrition advises against using components such as dextrose, fructose, glucose, sucrose, and corn syrup.

White flour contains a lot of simple carbs, which cause a lot of insulin to be released.

While it's important to learn what to avoid in a PCOS dessert, here's what to include:

Ingredients for PCOS-friendly desserts

There is a list of PCOS-friendly baking ingredients that you can use, which includes:

- Alternatives to milk
- Substitutes for sugar
- Alternatives to flour

Alternatives to milk

Almond milk, coconut milk, oat milk, and other milk substitutes are available. Simply searching for a PCOS cake recipe that uses any of these milk replacements online is an easy way to locate one. For example, searching for "almond milk chocolate cake recipe" yields a plethora of dairy-free chocolate cake recipes.

Sugar substitutes

Natural and artificial sweeteners are sugar substitutes. BBC Food suggests sugar substitutes for desserts: Honey and maple syrup are examples of natural sugars. Erythritol and Xylitol are sugar alcohols. Stevia, agave nectar, and rice malt syrup are examples of sweet extracts.

When choosing a sugar substitute, extensively research your options. I discovered a lot of information about the potential dangers of non-nutritive sweeteners like Stevia while writing this piece. According to the journal Nutrients, some evidence suggests that non-nutritive sweeteners can disrupt the gut microbiome.

"Consumers must be aware that, contrary to popular belief, replacing natural sugar with NAS is beneficial to their health, and there is growing evidence that NAS is involved in the development of metabolic abnormalities. "During my investigation, I also came across a couple of recipes that included rice malt sugar. However, rice malt syrup may not be the best sugar substitute. It not only raises blood sugar levels, but it may also contain significant doses of arsenic.

"Its high GI, lack of nutrients, and arsenic contamination risk are significant drawbacks." Rice syrup appears to be largely detrimental, even if it is fructose-free. "Coconut sugar could also work as an alternative. This chocolate cake recipe calls for either coconut sugar or honey.

Substitutes for flour

Whole wheat flour, almond flour, and coconut flour are all good alternatives to white flour. If you use a flour replacement, keep in mind that you will most likely need to modify the recipe in some way. Consider the healthy chocolate recipe that calls for whole wheat flour. To cover a "wheaty taste," cocoa powder, oil, and sugar are used.

15 RECIPES

Berry Chia Seed Pudding

Prep Time:	**Chill Time:**	**Serving Size:**
10 minutes	4 hours or overnight	Serves 2 persons

INGREDIENTS:

- 1 cup of non-sweetened almond milk (or any milk of your choice)
- 1/4 cup chia seeds
- 1 tablespoon honey (or maple syrup for a vegan option)
- 1/2 teaspoon vanilla extract
- 1/2 cup mixed berries (strawberries, blueberries, raspberries)
- Optional toppings: additional berries, shredded coconut, chopped nuts

INSTRUCTIONS:

- In a mixing bowl, whisk together the almond milk, chia seeds, honey (or maple syrup), and vanilla extract until well combined.
- Let the mixture sit for a few minutes, and then whisk again to prevent clumping.
- Cover the bowl with plastic wrap or a lid and refrigerate for at least 4 hours or preferably overnight, to allow the chia seeds to gel and thicken the pudding.
- Before serving, give the chia seed pudding a good stir to ensure a smooth and creamy texture.
- Divide the chia seed pudding into serving bowls or glasses.
- Top the pudding with mixed berries and any desired toppings like additional berries, shredded coconut, or chopped nuts for added flavor and texture.
- Enjoy the delicious and nutrient-rich berry chia seed pudding as a delightful breakfast or a healthy dessert.

NUTRITIONAL FACTS (PER SERVING):

- Calories: approximately 200 kcal
- Carbohydrates: 20g
- Protein: 6g
- Fat: 10g
- Fiber: 12g

Almond Flour Chocolate Chip Cookies

Prep Time:	Bake Time:	Serving Size:
15 minutes	10-12 minutes	Makes about 12 cookies

INGREDIENTS:

- 1 cup almond flour
- 1/4 cup coconut oil, melted
- 1/4 cup maple syrup
- 1 teaspoon vanilla extract
- 1/4 teaspoon baking soda
- Pinch of salt
- 1/3 cup dark chocolate chips (or any chocolate chips of your choice)

INSTRUCTIONS:

- Get your oven warming up to 350°F (175°C). Line a baking sheet with parchment paper.
- In a mixing bowl, combine almond flour, melted coconut oil, maple syrup, vanilla extract, baking soda, and a pinch of salt. Mix until the dough comes together.
- Fold in the dark chocolate chips.
- Using a tablespoon or cookie scoop, portion the cookie dough onto the prepared baking sheet, leaving enough space between each cookie.
- Gently flatten the cookie dough with the back of a fork or your fingers.
- Bake the cookies in the preheated oven for 10-12 mins till they are lightly golden around the edges.
- Let the cookies cool on the baking sheet for a few minutes before transferring them to a wire rack to cool completely.
- Once cooled, store the almond flour chocolate chip cookies in an airtight container for freshness.
- Enjoy the delightful and healthier almond flour chocolate chip cookies as a guilt-free treat.

NUTRITIONAL FACTS (PER COOKIE):

- Calories: approximately 150 kcal
- Carbohydrates: 10g
- Protein: 3g
- Fat: 12g
- Fiber: 2g

Greek Yogurt Parfait with Berries and Granola

Prep Time:	**Serving Size:**
10 minutes	Serves 2 persons

INGREDIENTS:

- 1 cup Greek yogurt
- 1 cup mixed berries (strawberries, blueberries, raspberries)
- 1/2 cup granola (homemade or store-bought)
- Optional toppings: drizzle of honey, chopped nuts, fresh mint leaves

INSTRUCTIONS:

- In a glass or serving bowl, layer the Greek yogurt, mixed berries, and granola in alternating layers.
- Repeat the layering until you use up all the ingredients, ending with a layer of berries on top.
- If desired, drizzle a little honey over the top layer for added sweetness.
- Sprinkle chopped nuts over the parfait for extra crunch and nutrition.
- Garnish with fresh mint leaves for a pop of color and freshness.
- Serve the Greek yogurt parfait with berries and granola as a delightful and nutritious breakfast or a wholesome dessert.

NUTRITIONAL FACTS (PER SERVING):

- Calories: approximately 300 kcal
- Carbohydrates: 35g
- Protein: 15g
- Fat: 10g
- Fiber: 5g

Baked Apples with Cinnamon

Prep Time:	**Bake Time:**	**Serving Size:**
10 minutes	20-25 minutes	Serves 2 persons

INGREDIENTS:

- 2 large apples (your favorite variety), washed and cored
- 2 tablespoons unsalted butter (or coconut oil for a vegan option)
- 2 tablespoons honey (or maple syrup for a vegan option)
- 1 teaspoon ground cinnamon
- Pinch of nutmeg (optional)

INSTRUCTIONS:

- Get your oven warming up to 375°F (190°C). Line a baking dish with parchment paper.
- Cut the top off each cored apple, creating a well for the filling.
- In a small bowl, mix the butter (or coconut oil), honey (or maple syrup), ground cinnamon, and a pinch of nutmeg (if using).
- Stuff each apple with the cinnamon mixture, making sure the well is filled.
- Place the stuffed apples in the prepared baking dish.
- Bake the apples in the preheated oven for 20-25 mins till they are tender and slightly caramelized.
- Remove the baked apples from the oven and let them cool slightly before serving.
- Enjoy the warm and comforting baked apples with cinnamon as a delightful and healthier dessert option.

NUTRITIONAL FACTS (PER SERVING):

- Calories: approximately 200 kcal
- Carbohydrates: 40g
- Protein: 1g
- Fat: 5g
- Fiber: 6g

Coconut and Berry Frozen Yogurt

Prep Time:	**Freeze Time:**	**Serving Size:**
10 minutes	4 hours or overnight	Serves 2 persons

INGREDIENTS:

- 2 cups frozen mixed berries (strawberries, blueberries, raspberries)
- 1 cup Greek yogurt
- 1/4 cup unsweetened coconut milk
- 2 tablespoons honey (or maple syrup for a vegan option)
- 1/4 cup shredded coconut (unsweetened)
- Fresh mint leaves for garnish

INSTRUCTIONS:

- In a blender or food processor, combine frozen mixed berries, Greek yogurt, coconut milk, and honey (or maple syrup).
- Blend the ingredients until you achieve a smooth and creamy consistency.
- Taste the frozen yogurt and adjust the sweetness with more honey or maple syrup if needed.
- Fold the shredded coconut into the frozen yogurt for added texture and flavor.
- Pour the frozen yogurt mixture into a freezer-safe container or individual serving dishes.
- Cover the container with a lid or plastic wrap and freeze the coconut and berry frozen yogurt for at least 4 hours or preferably overnight to firm up.
- Before serving, let the frozen yogurt sit at room temperature for a few minutes to soften slightly.
- Garnish with fresh mint leaves for a burst of color and freshness.
- Enjoy the delightful and creamy coconut and berry frozen yogurt as a refreshing and guilt-free frozen treat.

NUTRITIONAL FACTS (PER SERVING):

- Calories: approximately 250 kcal
- Carbohydrates: 30g
- Protein: 10g
- Fat: 10g
- Fiber: 6g

Dark Chocolate Almond Clusters

Prep Time:	Chill Time:	Serving Size:
10 minutes	30 minutes	Makes about 12 clusters

INGREDIENTS:

- 1 cup dark chocolate chips (70% cocoa or higher)
- 1 cup roasted almonds
- Sea salt flakes (optional)

INSTRUCTIONS:

- Line a baking sheet with parchment paper or a silicone mat.
- In a microwave-safe bowl, melt the dark chocolate chips in 30-second intervals, stirring in between, until fully melted and smooth.
- Add the roasted almonds to the melted chocolate, stirring until all almonds are coated.
- Using a spoon or fork, scoop clusters of the chocolate-coated almonds onto the prepared baking sheet, leaving some space between each cluster.
- Sprinkle a pinch of sea salt flakes over the clusters if desired.
- Chill the almond clusters in the refrigerator for about 30 mins till the chocolate is fully set.
- Once the clusters are firm, remove them from the refrigerator and transfer them to an airtight container for storage.
- Enjoy the irresistible and indulgent dark chocolate almond clusters as a delectable treat or a thoughtful gift.

NUTRITIONAL FACTS (PER CLUSTER):

- Calories: approximately 100 kcal
- Carbohydrates: 9g
- Protein: 2g
- Fat: 7g
- Fiber: 2g

Banana Almond Butter Ice Cream

Prep Time:	**Freeze Time:**	**Serving Size:**
10 minutes	4 hours or overnight	Serves 2-3 persons

INGREDIENTS:

- 4 ripe bananas, peeled and sliced
- 1/4 cup almond butter
- 1/4 cup unsweetened almond milk (or any milk of your choice)
- 1 teaspoon vanilla extract
- Optional toppings: chopped almonds, dark chocolate shavings

INSTRUCTIONS:

- Place the sliced bananas in a single layer on a baking sheet lined with parchment paper or aluminum foil.
- Freeze the banana slices for at least 4 hours or preferably overnight until they are solid.
- In a blender or food processor, combine the frozen banana slices, almond butter, almond milk, and vanilla extract.
- Blend the mixture until you achieve a smooth and creamy consistency, similar to soft-serve ice cream.
- If the mixture is too thick, you can add a little more almond milk to help with blending.
- Transfer the banana almond butter ice cream to a freezer-safe container and freeze for an additional 1-2 hours for a firmer texture.
- Serve the delightful and guilt-free banana almond butter ice cream with your favorite toppings, such as chopped almonds or dark chocolate shavings.

NUTRITIONAL FACTS (PER SERVING, WITHOUT TOPPINGS):

- Calories: approximately 200 kcal
- Carbohydrates: 30g
- Protein: 4g
- Fat: 9g
- Fiber: 5g

Dark Chocolate Avocado Mousse

Prep Time:	Chill Time:	Serving Size:
15 minutes	2 hours	Serves 2-3 persons

INGREDIENTS:

- 2 ripe avocados, peeled and pitted
- 1/4 cup unsweetened cocoa powder
- 1/4 cup honey or maple syrup
- 1/4 cup almond milk (or any milk of your choice)
- 1 teaspoon vanilla extract
- Pinch of salt
- Optional toppings: whipped cream, dark chocolate curls

INSTRUCTIONS:

- In a blender or food processor, combine the peeled and pitted avocados, cocoa powder, honey (or maple syrup), almond milk, vanilla extract, and a pinch of salt.
- Blend the mixture until you achieve a smooth and creamy mousse consistency.
- Taste the mousse and adjust the sweetness with more honey or maple syrup if needed.
- Transfer the dark chocolate avocado mousse to individual serving dishes or a large bowl.
- Cover the mousse and refrigerate for at least 2 hours to chill and set.
- Before serving, garnish the dark chocolate avocado mousse with a dollop of whipped cream and dark chocolate curls for an elegant presentation.
- Enjoy the luscious and healthier dark chocolate avocado mousse as a delightful and indulgent dessert.

NUTRITIONAL FACTS (PER SERVING, WITHOUT TOPPINGS):

- Calories: approximately 250 kcal
- Carbohydrates: 25g
- Protein: 4g
- Fat: 16g
- Fiber: 9g

Peach and Raspberry Crumble

Prep Time:	Bake Time:	Serving Size:
15 minutes	30-35 minutes	Serves 4-6 persons

INGREDIENTS:

- 4 ripe peaches, peeled and sliced
- 1 cup fresh raspberries
- 2 tablespoons honey or maple syrup
- 1 teaspoon lemon juice
- 1/2 cup old-fashioned rolled oats
- 1/4 cup almond flour
- 2 tablespoons coconut oil, melted
- 2 tablespoons honey or maple syrup
- 1/4 teaspoon ground cinnamon
- Pinch of salt
- Optional toppings: vanilla ice cream, whipped cream

INSTRUCTIONS:

- Get your oven warming up to 350°F (175°C). Grease a baking dish with coconut oil or use a non-stick spray.
- In a mixing bowl, combine the sliced peaches, fresh raspberries, honey (or maple syrup), and lemon juice. Toss until the fruit is well coated.
- Transfer the peach and raspberry mixture to the greased baking dish, spreading it out in an even layer.
- In another bowl, mix the old-fashioned rolled oats, almond flour, melted coconut oil, honey (or maple syrup), ground cinnamon, and a pinch of salt until crumbly.
- Sprinkle the oat and almond crumble mixture evenly over the fruit in the baking dish.
- Bake the peach and raspberry crumble in the preheated oven for 30-35 mins till the topping is golden, and the fruit is bubbling.
- Remove the crumble from the oven and let it cool slightly before serving.
- Serve the delectable peach and raspberry crumble warm, topped with a scoop of vanilla ice cream or a dollop of whipped cream.

NUTRITIONAL FACTS (PER SERVING, WITHOUT TOPPINGS):

- Calories: approximately 200 kcal
- Carbohydrates: 30g
- Protein: 3g
- Fat: 8g
- Fiber: 5g

Healthy Pumpkin Bread

Prep Time:	Bake Time:	Serving Size:
15 minutes	50-55 minutes	Makes 1 loaf (8-10 slices)

INGREDIENTS:

- 1 3/4 cups whole wheat flour
- 1 teaspoon baking soda
- 1/2 teaspoon baking powder
- 1/2 teaspoon salt
- 1 teaspoon ground cinnamon
- 1/2 teaspoon ground nutmeg
- 1/4 teaspoon ground cloves
- 1 cup pumpkin puree (canned or homemade)
- 1/2 cup honey or maple syrup
- 1/3 cup unsweetened applesauce
- 1/4 cup coconut oil, melted
- 2 large eggs
- 1 teaspoon vanilla extract
- 1/2 cup chopped walnuts or pecans (optional)

INSTRUCTIONS:

- Get your oven warming up to 350°F (175°C). Grease a 9x5-inch loaf pan with coconut oil, or use parchment paper to line the bottom and sides.
- In a large mixing bowl, whisk together the whole wheat flour, baking soda, baking powder, salt, ground cinnamon, ground nutmeg, and ground cloves.
- In a separate bowl, mix the pumpkin puree, honey (or maple syrup), unsweetened applesauce, melted coconut oil, eggs, and vanilla extract until well combined.
- Pour the wet ingredients into the dry ingredients, stirring until just combined. Do not overmix.
- If desired, fold in the chopped walnuts or pecans into the batter for added crunch and flavor.
- Pour the pumpkin bread batter into the prepared loaf pan, spreading it out evenly.
- Bake the healthy pumpkin bread in the preheated oven for 50-55 mins till a toothpick inserted into the center comes out clean.
- Remove the bread from the oven and let it cool in the pan for about 10 minutes before transferring it to a wire rack to cool completely.
- Once cooled, slice the healthy pumpkin bread into 8-10 slices.
- Enjoy the moist and flavorful pumpkin bread as a satisfying breakfast or a delightful snack.

NUTRITIONAL FACTS (PER SLICE, WITHOUT NUTS):

- Calories: approximately 200 kcal
- Carbohydrates: 30g
- Protein: 4g
- Fat: 8g
- Fiber: 3g

Oatmeal Raisin Cookies

Prep Time:	Bake Time:	Serving Size:
15 minutes	10-12 minutes	Makes about 18 cookies

INGREDIENTS:

- 1 cup old-fashioned rolled oats
- 3/4 cup whole wheat flour
- 1/2 teaspoon baking soda
- 1/2 teaspoon ground cinnamon
- 1/4 teaspoon salt
- 1/2 cup unsalted butter, softened
- 1/2 cup brown sugar
- 1/4 cup granulated sugar
- 1 large egg
- 1 teaspoon vanilla extract
- 1/2 cup raisins

INSTRUCTIONS:

- Get your oven warming up to 350°F (175°C). Line a baking sheet with parchment paper.
- In a mixing bowl, whisk together the rolled oats, whole wheat flour, baking soda, ground cinnamon, and salt.
- In a separate large bowl, cream the softened butter with brown sugar and granulated sugar until light and fluffy.
- Beat in the egg and vanilla extract until well combined.
- Gradually add the dry ingredients to the wet ingredients, mixing until just combined.
- Stir in the raisins until evenly distributed throughout the cookie dough.
- Using a spoon or cookie scoop, drop tablespoons of dough onto the prepared baking sheet, leaving enough space between each cookie.
- Flatten each cookie slightly with the back of the spoon or your fingers.
- Bake the oatmeal raisin cookies in the preheated oven for 10-12 mins till the edges are golden brown.
- Remove the cookies from the oven and let them cool on the baking sheet for a few minutes before transferring them to a wire rack to cool completely.
- Enjoy the chewy and flavorful oatmeal raisin cookies as a delightful snack or a treat with your favorite beverage.

NUTRITIONAL FACTS (PER COOKIE):

- Calories: approximately 120 kcal
- Carbohydrates: 15g
- Protein: 2g
- Fat: 6g
- Fiber: 1g

Strawberry Banana Nice Cream

Prep Time:	**Freeze Time:**	**Serving Size:**
5 minutes	4 hours or overnight	Serves 2-3 persons

INGREDIENTS:

- 2 ripe bananas, peeled and sliced
- 1 cup frozen strawberries
- 1/4 cup unsweetened almond milk (or any milk of your choice)
- Optional toppings: fresh strawberries, banana slices, shredded coconut

INSTRUCTIONS:

- Place the sliced bananas and frozen strawberries in a single layer on a baking sheet lined with parchment paper or aluminum foil.
- Freeze the fruit for at least 4 hours or preferably overnight until they are solid.
- In a blender or food processor, combine the frozen banana slices, frozen strawberries, and almond milk.
- Blend the mixture until you achieve a smooth and creamy consistency, similar to soft-serve ice cream.
- If the mixture is too thick, you can add a little more almond milk to help with blending.
- Transfer the strawberry banana nice cream to a freezer-safe container and freeze for an additional 1-2 hours for a firmer texture.
- Before serving, let the ice cream sit at room temperature for a few minutes to soften slightly.
- Serve the refreshing and naturally sweet strawberry banana nice cream with fresh strawberries, banana slices, and shredded coconut for a delightful and guilt-free dessert.

NUTRITIONAL FACTS (PER SERVING, WITHOUT TOPPINGS):

- Calories: approximately 100 kcal
- Carbohydrates: 25g
- Protein: 2g
- Fat: 0.5g
- Fiber: 4g

Blueberry and Almond Galette

Prep Time:	**Bake Time:**	**Serving Size:**
15 minutes	30-35 minutes	Serves 4-6 persons

INGREDIENTS:

- 1 sheet of store-bought puff pastry (thawed if frozen)
- 1 1/2 cups fresh blueberries
- 2 tablespoons granulated sugar
- 1 tablespoon cornstarch
- 1 tablespoon lemon juice
- 1/4 teaspoon almond extract (optional)
- 1 egg, beaten (for egg wash)
- 1 tablespoon sliced almonds
- Honey or maple syrup for drizzling (optional)

INSTRUCTIONS:

- Get your oven warming up to 375°F (190°C). Line a baking sheet with parchment paper.
- In a mixing bowl, gently toss the fresh blueberries with granulated sugar, cornstarch, lemon juice, and almond extract (if using).
- Unroll the sheet of puff pastry onto the prepared baking sheet.
- Spoon the blueberry mixture onto the center of the puff pastry, leaving about 2 inches of border around the edges.
- Fold the edges of the puff pastry over the blueberries, pleating as you go to create a rustic galette shape.
- Brush the edges of the pastry with the beaten egg for a golden finish.
- Sprinkle sliced almonds over the top of the blueberries.
- Bake the blueberry and almond galette in the preheated oven for 30-35 mins till the pastry is golden, and the blueberries are bubbling.
- Remove the galette from the oven and let it cool slightly before serving.
- Drizzle honey or maple syrup over the galette if desired for added sweetness.
- Serve the delectable blueberry and almond galette warm, on its own or with a scoop of vanilla ice cream.

NUTRITIONAL FACTS (PER SERVING, WITHOUT DRIZZLE OR ICE CREAM):

- Calories: approximately 250 kcal
- Carbohydrates: 25g
- Protein: 3g
- Fat: 16g
- Fiber: 3g

Raspberry Chia Jam Thumbprint Cookies

Prep Time:	**Bake Time:**	**Chill Time:**	**Serving Size:**
15 minutes	10-12 minutes	30 minutes (for jam)	Makes about 18 cookies

INGREDIENTS:

- 1 cup whole wheat flour
- 1/2 cup unsalted butter, softened
- 1/4 cup honey or maple syrup
- 1/2 teaspoon vanilla extract
- 1/4 teaspoon salt
- 1/4 cup raspberry chia jam (store-bought or homemade)

INSTRUCTIONS:

- In a mixing bowl, combine whole wheat flour, softened butter, honey (or maple syrup), vanilla extract, and salt until a soft dough forms.
- Shape the dough into a ball, cover with plastic wrap, and refrigerate for 30 minutes to firm up.
- Get your oven warming up to 350°F (175°C). Line a baking sheet with parchment paper.
- Roll the chilled cookie dough into 1-inch balls and place them on the prepared baking sheet, leaving enough space between each cookie.
- Use your thumb or the back of a teaspoon to make an indentation in the center of each cookie.
- Fill each indentation with a small spoonful of raspberry chia jam.
- Bake the raspberry chia jam thumbprint cookies in the preheated oven for 10-12 mins till the edges are lightly golden.
- Remove the cookies from the oven and let them cool on the baking sheet for a few minutes before transferring them to a wire rack to cool completely.
- Enjoy the wholesome and fruity raspberry chia jam thumbprint cookies as a delightful treat with a cup of tea or coffee.

NUTRITIONAL FACTS (PER COOKIE):

- Calories: approximately 100 kcal
- Carbohydrates: 10g
- Protein: 2g
- Fat: 6g
- Fiber: 1g

Lemon and Poppy Seed Muffins

Prep Time:	Bake Time:	Serving Size:
15 minutes	18-20 minutes	Makes 12 muffins

INGREDIENTS:

- 1 3/4 cups all-purpose flour
- 1/2 cup granulated sugar
- 2 teaspoons baking powder
- 1/4 teaspoon baking soda
- 1/4 teaspoon salt
- 1 tablespoon poppy seeds
- Zest of 1 lemon
- 1/2 cup unsalted butter, melted and cooled
- 1/2 cup plain Greek yogurt
- 1/4 cup fresh lemon juice
- 2 large eggs
- 1 teaspoon vanilla extract
- Optional glaze: 1/2 cup powdered sugar, 1 tablespoon fresh lemon juice

INSTRUCTIONS:

- Get your oven warming up to 375°F (190°C). Line a muffin tin with paper liners or grease the muffin cups.
- In a large mixing bowl, whisk together the all-purpose flour, granulated sugar, baking powder, baking soda, salt, poppy seeds, and lemon zest.
- In a separate bowl, mix the melted butter, Greek yogurt, fresh lemon juice, eggs, and vanilla extract until well combined.
- Pour the wet ingredients into the dry ingredients, stirring until just combined. Do not overmix; a few lumps are okay.
- Divide the muffin batter evenly among the muffin cups, filling each about two-thirds full.
- Bake the lemon and poppy seed muffins in the preheated oven for 18-20 mins till a toothpick inserted into the center of a muffin comes out clean.
- Remove the muffins from the oven and let them cool in the muffin tin for a few minutes before transferring them to a wire rack to cool completely.
- If desired, whisk together the powdered sugar and fresh lemon juice to make a simple glaze. Drizzle the glaze over the cooled muffins for extra sweetness and tanginess.

- Enjoy the light and zesty lemon and poppy seed muffins as a delightful breakfast or a tasty snack.

NUTRITIONAL FACTS (PER MUFFIN, WITHOUT GLAZE):

- Calories: approximately 180 kcal
- Carbohydrates: 24g
- Protein: 3g
- Fat: 8g
- Fiber: 1g

CHAPTER 8

PCOS-FRIENDLY BEVERAGES

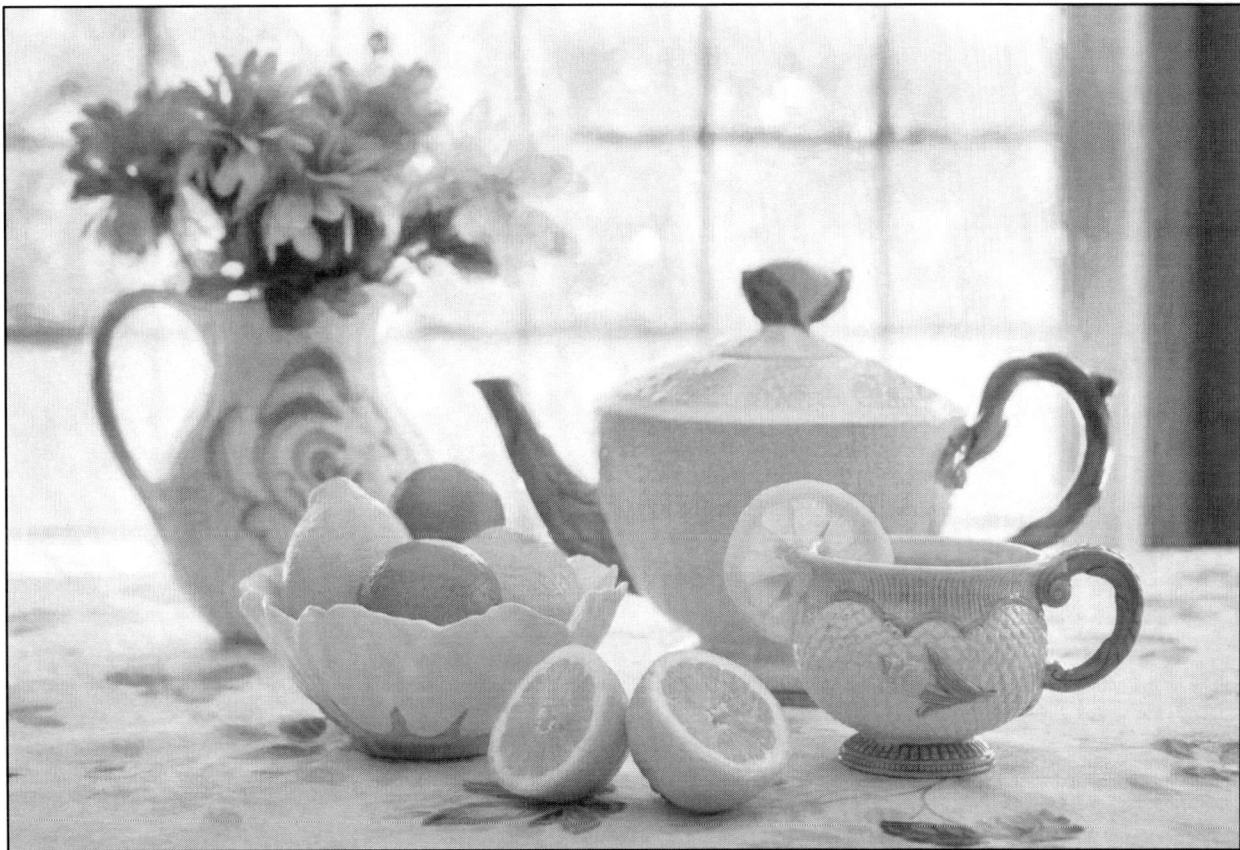

One crucial aspect of managing PCOS through diet is to make mindful choices regarding the beverages we consume. Many commercial drinks are laden with added sugars, artificial flavors, and other unhealthy ingredients that can worsen PCOS symptoms. In this chapter, we will explore 15 PCOS-friendly beverage recipes that are not only delicious but also support hormonal balance and overall well-being.

15 RECIPES

Berry Antioxidant Smoothie

Prep Time:

5 minutes

Serving Size:

Serves 1 person

INGREDIENTS:

- 1 cup mixed berries (strawberries, blueberries, raspberries)
- 1 ripe banana
- 1/2 cup Greek yogurt
- 1 tablespoon honey
- 1/2 cup almond milk (or any milk of your choice)
- 1 tablespoon chia seeds (optional)
- Ice cubes (optional)

INSTRUCTIONS:

- In a blender, combine the mixed berries, ripe banana, Greek yogurt, honey, and almond milk.
- If desired, add chia seeds for added nutrition and thickness to the smoothie.
- Blend all the ingredients until smooth and creamy. If you prefer a colder smoothie, you can add some ice cubes as well.
- Pour the berry antioxidant smoothie into a glass and serve immediately.

- Enjoy the delicious and refreshing smoothie packed with antioxidants and nutrients.

NUTRITIONAL FACTS:

- Calories: approximately 300 kcal
- Carbohydrates: 55g
- Protein: 12g
- Fat: 6g
- Fiber: 9g

Detox Green Juice

Prep Time:	**Serving Size:**
10 minutes	Serves 1 person

INGREDIENTS:

- 2 cups fresh spinach
- 1 cucumber
- 1 green apple
- 1 lemon, peeled
- 1-inch piece of fresh ginger
- 1 cup water
- Ice cubes (optional)

INSTRUCTIONS:

- Wash all the produce thoroughly.
- Cut the cucumber and green apple into smaller pieces for easier blending.
- In a juicer or a high-speed blender, add the fresh spinach, cucumber, green apple, peeled lemon, and fresh ginger.
- Add water to help with blending and extracting the juice.
- Blend all the ingredients until smooth and well combined.
- If desired, add ice cubes to the juice for a refreshing and chilled detox drink.
- Pour the green juice into a glass and serve immediately.
- Enjoy the nutrient-packed and cleansing detox green juice to kickstart your day.

NUTRITIONAL FACTS:

- Calories: approximately 150 kcal
- Carbohydrates: 36g
- Protein: 4g
- Fat: 1g
- Fiber: 10g

Cinnamon and Honey Infused Water

Prep Time:	Chill Time:	Serving Size:
5 minutes	1 hour	Serves 1 person

INGREDIENTS:

- 1 cup water
- 1 cinnamon stick
- 1 tablespoon honey
- Ice cubes (optional)

INSTRUCTIONS:

- In a glass or jar, add the water and the cinnamon stick.
- Let the cinnamon stick infuse the water for at least 1 hour to impart its flavor and health benefits.
- After the infusion time, remove the cinnamon stick from the water.
- Stir in the honey until it dissolves completely in the infused water.
- If desired, add ice cubes to the infused water for a refreshing drink.
- Stir the water once again before drinking to evenly distribute the cinnamon and honey flavors.

- Sip on the soothing and naturally sweet cinnamon and honey-infused water as a flavorful and healthy alternative to plain water.

NUTRITIONAL FACTS:

- Calories: approximately 50 kcal
- Carbohydrates: 13g
- Protein: 0g
- Fat: 0g
- Fiber: 0g

Lemon Ginger Herbal Tea

Prep Time:	Steep Time:	Serving Size:
5 minutes	5 minutes	Serves 1 person

INGREDIENTS:

- 1 cup water
- 1-inch piece of fresh ginger, sliced
- 1 tablespoon fresh lemon juice
- 1 teaspoon honey (optional)

INSTRUCTIONS:

- In a small saucepan, bring the water to a boil.
- Add the sliced fresh ginger to the boiling water and let it simmer for about 3-5 minutes to infuse the ginger flavor.
- Remove the saucepan from the heat and strain the ginger pieces, leaving only the ginger-infused water.
- Stir in the fresh lemon juice and honey (if using) into the ginger-infused water.
- Pour the lemon ginger herbal tea into a cup and serve immediately.
- Savor the soothing and aromatic lemon ginger herbal tea, perfect for a relaxing and comforting moment.

NUTRITIONAL FACTS:

- Calories: approximately 10 kcal
- Carbohydrates: 3g
- Protein: 0g
- Fat: 0g
- Fiber: 0g

Turmeric and Black Pepper Tea

Prep Time:	Steep Time:	Serving Size:
5 minutes	5 minutes	Serves 1 person

INGREDIENTS:

- 1 cup water
- 1 teaspoon ground turmeric
- 1/4 teaspoon ground black pepper
- 1 teaspoon honey (optional)
- 1 tablespoon coconut milk (or any milk of your choice)

INSTRUCTIONS:

- In a small saucepan, bring the water to a boil.
- Stir in the ground turmeric and ground black pepper into the boiling water.
- Let the turmeric and black pepper steep in the water for about 3-5 minutes to infuse the flavors.
- Remove the saucepan from the heat.
- Stir in honey (if using) and coconut milk into the turmeric and black pepper tea.
- Pour the turmeric and black pepper tea into a cup and serve immediately.
- Enjoy the warming and spiced turmeric and black pepper tea, which is known for its potential health benefits.

NUTRITIONAL FACTS:

- Calories: approximately 20 kcal
- Carbohydrates: 4g
- Protein: 0g
- Fat: 1g
- Fiber: 1g

Chia Seed Hydrating Drink

Prep Time:	Chill Time:	Serving Size:
5 minutes	1-2 hours	Serves 1 person
	(for chia seeds to hydrate)	

INGREDIENTS:

- 1 cup coconut water (or plain water)
- 1 tablespoon chia seeds
- 1 tablespoon fresh lemon or lime juice
- 1 teaspoon honey (optional)

INSTRUCTIONS:

- In a glass or jar, mix the coconut water (or plain water) with chia seeds.
- Stir the mixture well to ensure the chia seeds are evenly distributed.
- Let the chia seeds hydrate in the liquid for at least 1-2 hours. You can also prepare this drink in advance and leave it in the refrigerator overnight for a refreshing beverage the next day.
- After the chia seeds have hydrated, stir in the fresh lemon or lime juice and honey (if using) to add a hint of citrus flavor and sweetness.
- Give the drink a final stir before serving.
- Sip on the chia seed hydrating drink for a refreshing and hydrating boost, especially on a hot day.

NUTRITIONAL FACTS:

- Calories: approximately 60 kcal
- Carbohydrates: 8g
- Protein: 2g
- Fat: 3g
- Fiber: 4g

Pomegranate and Lime Iced Tea

Prep Time:	Chill Time:	Serving Size:
10 minutes	2-3 hours (for tea to cool)	Serves 2-3 persons

INGREDIENTS:

- 2 cups water
- 2 black tea bags (or any tea of your choice)
- 1/2 cup pomegranate juice (100% pure)
- Juice of 1 lime
- 2 tablespoons honey (adjust to taste)
- Ice cubes
- Fresh pomegranate arils and lime slices for garnish

INSTRUCTIONS:

- In a saucepan, bring the water to a boil.
- Remove the saucepan from the heat and add the tea bags. Let the tea steep for about 5 minutes to reach the desired strength.
- Remove the tea bags and let the tea cool to room temperature.
- Once the tea has cooled, stir in the pomegranate juice, fresh lime juice, and honey until well combined.
- Chill the pomegranate and lime iced tea in the refrigerator for 2-3 hrs. till it is thoroughly chilled.
- Before serving, add ice cubes to glasses and pour the iced tea over the ice.
- Garnish the glasses with fresh pomegranate arils and lime slices for a beautiful presentation.
- Savor the refreshing and tangy pomegranate and lime iced tea as a delightful and colorful beverage.

NUTRITIONAL FACTS (PER SERVING):

- Calories: approximately 80 kcal
- Carbohydrates: 21g
- Protein: 1g
- Fat: 0g
- Fiber: 1g

Almond Milk Matcha Latte

Prep Time:

5 minutes

Serving Size:

Serves 1 person

INGREDIENTS:

- 1 teaspoon matcha green tea powder
- 1 tablespoon hot water
- 1 cup of non-sweetened almond milk (or any milk of your choice)
- 1 teaspoon honey or maple syrup (adjust to taste)

INSTRUCTIONS:

- In a bowl, whisk the matcha green tea powder with hot water until it becomes a smooth and vibrant green paste.
- In a saucepan, heat the almond milk over medium heat until it is steaming hot. Be careful not to boil the milk.
- Pour the hot almond milk into a cup.
- Stir in the matcha paste into the hot almond milk until it is well blended.
- Sweeten the almond milk matcha latte with honey or maple syrup, adjusting the sweetness to your preference.
- Give the latte a final stir before serving.

- Sip on the creamy and earthy almond milk matcha latte as a soothing and energizing beverage.

NUTRITIONAL FACTS:

- Calories: approximately 60 kcal
- Carbohydrates: 6g
- Protein: 2g
- Fat: 4g
- Fiber: 1g

Green Apple and Spinach Smoothie

Prep Time:

5 minutes

Serving Size:

Serves 1 person

INGREDIENTS:

- 1 green apple, cored and chopped
- 1 cup fresh spinach leaves
- 1/2 cup plain Greek yogurt
- 1/2 cup unsweetened almond milk (or any milk of your choice)
- 1 tablespoon honey or maple syrup (adjust to taste)
- Ice cubes (optional)

INSTRUCTIONS:

- In a blender, combine the chopped green apple, fresh spinach leaves, plain Greek yogurt, and unsweetened almond milk.
- If desired, add honey or maple syrup to sweeten the smoothie according to your taste preference.
- Blend all the ingredients until smooth and creamy. If you prefer a colder smoothie, you can add some ice cubes as well.
- Pour the green apple and spinach smoothie into a glass and serve immediately.

- Enjoy the nutrient-packed and refreshing green smoothie, which is perfect for a healthy start to your day.

NUTRITIONAL FACTS:

- Calories: approximately 150 kcal
- Carbohydrates: 24g
- Protein: 7g
- Fat: 4g
- Fiber: 5g

Golden Milk (Turmeric Milk)

Prep Time:

5 minutes

Serving Size:

Serves 1 person

INGREDIENTS:

- 1 cup of non-sweetened almond milk (or any milk of your choice)
- 1 teaspoon ground turmeric
- 1/4 teaspoon ground cinnamon
- Pinch of ground black pepper
- 1 tablespoon honey or maple syrup (adjust to taste)
- 1/2 teaspoon coconut oil (optional)

INSTRUCTIONS:

- ◆ In a small saucepan, heat the unsweetened almond milk over medium heat until it is steaming hot. Be careful not to boil the milk.
- ◆ Stir in the ground turmeric, ground cinnamon, and a pinch of ground black pepper into the hot almond milk.
- ◆ If desired, add honey or maple syrup to sweeten the golden milk according to your taste preference.
- ◆ For an added creamy texture and taste, you can stir coconut oil into the golden milk.

- ◆ Give the golden milk a final stir before serving.
- ◆ Sip on the warm and aromatic golden milk, which is known for its potential health benefits and soothing properties.

NUTRITIONAL FACTS:

- Calories: approximately 100 kcal
- Carbohydrates: 15g
- Protein: 2g
- Fat: 4g
- Fiber: 2g

Iced Raspberry Leaf Tea

Prep Time:	Chill Time:	Serving Size:
5 minutes	2-3 hours (for tea to cool)	Serves 2-3 persons

INGREDIENTS:

- 2 cups water
- 2 tablespoons dried raspberry leaves (or 4-5 fresh raspberry leaves)
- 1 tablespoon honey or maple syrup (adjust to taste)
- Ice cubes
- Fresh raspberries and mint leaves for garnish

INSTRUCTIONS:

- In a saucepan, bring the water to a boil.
- Remove the saucepan from the heat and add the dried raspberry leaves (or fresh raspberry leaves).
- Let the raspberry leaves steep in the water for about 5 minutes to infuse the tea.
- After steeping, strain the raspberry leaves from the tea.
- Stir in honey or maple syrup into the raspberry tea, adjusting the sweetness to your liking.
- Chill the raspberry leaf tea in the refrigerator for 2-3 hrs. till it is thoroughly chilled.
- Before serving, add ice cubes to glasses and pour the iced raspberry leaf tea over the ice.
- Garnish the glasses with fresh raspberries and mint leaves for a delightful touch.
- Sip on the refreshing and naturally fruity iced raspberry leaf tea, which is known for its potential health benefits.

NUTRITIONAL FACTS (PER SERVING):

- Calories: approximately 20 kcal
- Carbohydrates: 5g
- Protein: 0g
- Fat: 0g
- Fiber: 1g

Cucumber Mint Infused Water

Prep Time:	Chill Time:	Serving Size:
5 minutes	1-2 hours	Serves 1 person
	(for water to infuse)	

INGREDIENTS:

- 1 cup water
- 1/2 cucumber, sliced
- 5-6 fresh mint leaves
- Ice cubes

INSTRUCTIONS:

- In a glass or jar, add the water, sliced cucumber, and fresh mint leaves.
- Stir the ingredients gently to help release the flavors.
- Let the cucumber and mint infuse the water for at least 1-2 hours to enhance the taste.
- If desired, add ice cubes to the infused water for a refreshing drink.
- Give the water a gentle stir before serving.
- Sip on the cool and refreshing cucumber mint-infused water for a hydrating and invigorating experience.

NUTRITIONAL FACTS:

- Calories: approximately 0 kcal
- Carbohydrates: 0g
- Protein: 0g
- Fat: 0g
- Fiber: 0g

Chocolate Avocado Smoothie

Prep Time:

5 minutes

Serving Size:

Serves 1 person

INGREDIENTS:

- 1 ripe avocado, peeled and pitted
- 1 ripe banana
- 1 cup of non-sweetened almond milk (or any milk of your choice)
- 2 tablespoons unsweetened cocoa powder
- 1 tablespoon honey or maple syrup (adjust to taste)
- Ice cubes (optional)

INSTRUCTIONS:

- In a blender, combine the ripe avocado, ripe banana, unsweetened almond milk, unsweetened cocoa powder, and honey or maple syrup.
- Blend all the ingredients until smooth and creamy. If you prefer a colder smoothie, you can add some ice cubes as well.
- Pour the chocolate avocado smoothie into a glass and serve immediately.

- Enjoy the rich and indulgent chocolate avocado smoothie, which offers a perfect balance of creaminess and chocolatey goodness.

NUTRITIONAL FACTS:

- Calories: approximately 300 kcal
- Carbohydrates: 40g
- Protein: 5g
- Fat: 18g
- Fiber: 12g

Hibiscus and Ginger Iced Tea

Prep Time:	**Chill Time:**	**Serving Size:**
5 minutes	2-3 hours (for tea to cool)	Serves 2-3 persons

INGREDIENTS:

- 2 cups water
- 2 tablespoons dried hibiscus flowers
- 1-inch piece of fresh ginger, sliced
- 1 tablespoon honey or maple syrup (adjust to taste)
- Ice cubes
- Fresh lemon slices and mint leaves for garnish

INSTRUCTIONS:

- In a saucepan, bring the water to a boil.
- Remove the saucepan from the heat and add the dried hibiscus flowers and sliced fresh ginger.
- Let the hibiscus and ginger steep in the water for about 5 minutes to infuse the tea.
- After steeping, strain the hibiscus flowers and ginger from the tea.
- Stir in honey or maple syrup into the hibiscus and ginger tea, adjusting the sweetness to your preference.
- Chill the hibiscus and ginger iced tea in the refrigerator for 2-3 hrs. till it is thoroughly chilled.
- Before serving, add ice cubes to glasses and pour the iced tea over the ice.
- Garnish the glasses with fresh lemon slices and mint leaves for a vibrant and refreshing presentation.
- Sip on the zesty and tangy hibiscus and ginger iced tea for a delightful and invigorating drink.

NUTRITIONAL FACTS (PER SERVING):

- Calories: approximately 10 kcal
- Carbohydrates: 2g
- Protein: 0g
- Fat: 0g
- Fiber: 0g

Fresh Squeezed Orange and Carrot Juice

Prep Time:	**Serving Size:**
10 minutes	Serves 1 person

INGREDIENTS:

- 2 large oranges, peeled and segmented
- 2 large carrots, washed and peeled
- Ice cubes (optional)

INSTRUCTIONS:

- Juice the oranges and carrots using a juicer or a blender with a fine-mesh strainer.
- If using a blender, blend the oranges and carrots until smooth, then strain the mixture through a fine-mesh strainer to remove any pulp.
- If desired, add ice cubes to the freshly squeezed juice for a chilled drink.
- Give the juice a final stir before serving.
- Sip on the vitamin-packed and naturally sweet orange and carrot juice for a refreshing and nourishing beverage.

NUTRITIONAL FACTS:

- Calories: approximately 120 kcal
- Carbohydrates: 28g
- Protein: 2g
- Fat: 0g
- Fiber: 4g

CHAPTER 9

MEAL PLANS AND WEEKLY MENUS

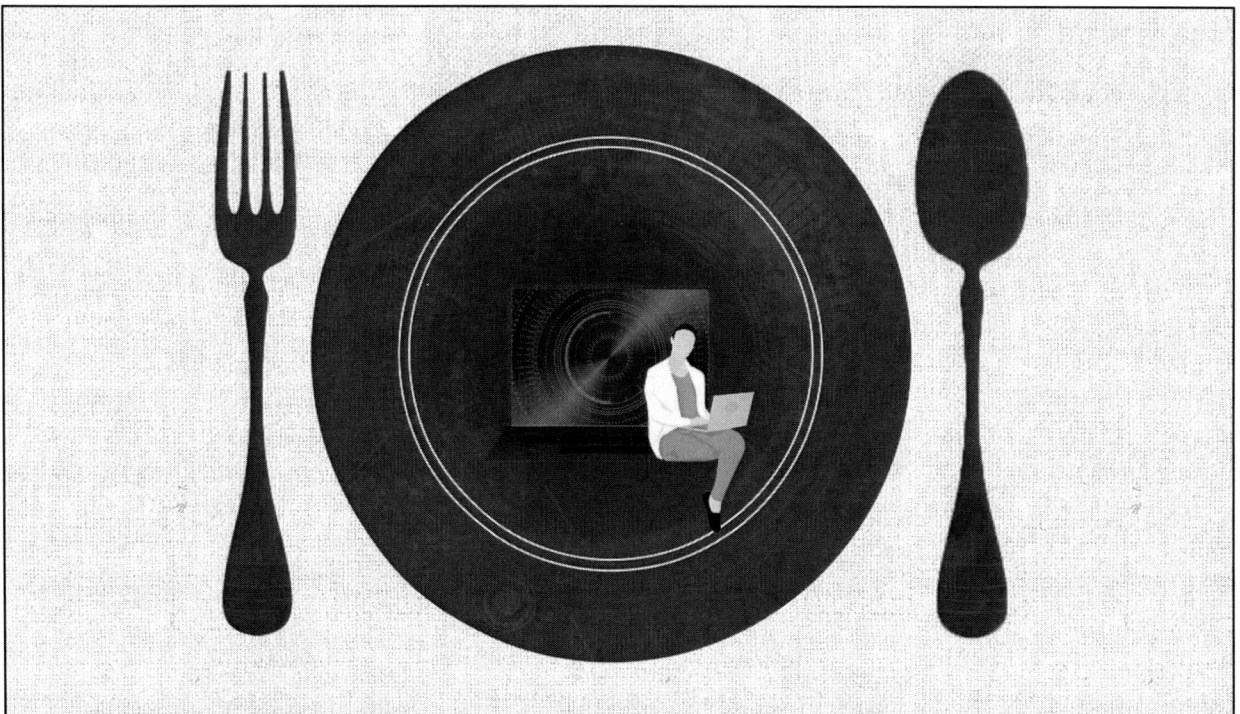

I n this chapter, we will delve into the significance of meal planning for PCOS patients and provide comprehensive insights into developing effective meal plans and weekly menus. We understand that starting on a new diet can be overwhelming, so we will begin with a 7-Day Meal Plan for Beginners. This plan will serve as an excellent foundation for those new to managing their PCOS through diet. Furthermore, we will discuss Seasonal Meal Planning Tips, highlighting the benefits of incorporating fresh, locally sourced produce into your diet. Finally, we will offer Weekly Menu Templates to help you streamline your meal preparation and ensure variety in your diet.

7-DAY MEAL PLAN FOR BEGINNERS

Day	Breakfast	Lunch	Dinner	Snack
Day 1	Berry Chia Seed Pudding	Grilled Salmon Salad with Lemon Vinaigrette	Hibiscus and Ginger Iced Tea	Almond Butter Energy Balls
Day 2	Oatmeal Raisin Cookies	Vegan Lentil Loaf with Tomato Glaze	Zucchini Noodles with Avocado Pesto	Baked Sweet Potato Chips
Day 3	Iced Raspberry Leaf Tea	Hearty Chicken and Vegetable Stew	Spaghetti Squash Pasta with Chunky Tomato Sauce	Spiced Roasted Chickpeas
Day 4	Chia Seed Hydrating Drink	Stuffed Acorn Squash with Wild Rice and Veggies	Black Bean and Corn Tacos	Spiced Roasted Chickpeas
Day 5	Lemon Herb Roasted Chicken with Brussels Sprouts	Green Apple and Spinach Smoothie	Baked Cod with Zesty Lemon Sauce	Fresh Squeezed Orange and Carrot Juice
Day 6	Chocolate Avocado Smoothie	Quinoa-Stuffed Bell Peppers	Lentil and Vegetable Curry	Greek Salad Skewers
Day 7	Golden Milk (Turmeric Milk)	Ratatouille with Quinoa	Tofu Pad Thai with Brown Rice Noodles	Apple Slices with Almond Butter

Please note that this is a sample meal plan and can be adjusted to fit your individual dietary preferences and needs. Remember to drink plenty of water throughout the day and listen to your body's hunger and fullness cues. Enjoy your delicious and nutritious meals!

SEASONAL MEAL PLANNING TIPS

Seasonal meal planning is an artful and sustainable approach to nourishing our bodies while savoring the ever-changing flavors nature has to offer. It involves tailoring our meals around the availability of fresh, locally grown ingredients during specific times of the year. This guide will take you through the intricacies of seasonal meal planning, exploring its numerous benefits, practical tips, and mouthwatering recipes that celebrate each season's bounty. From spring's vibrant greens to summer's luscious berries, autumn's hearty squashes, and winter's comforting stews, embracing seasonal eating not only delights the palate but also contributes to an eco-friendlier and more mindful lifestyle.

Benefits of Seasonal Meal Planning:

1. Improved Nutritional Value: Seasonal produce is harvested at its peak ripeness, delivering optimal flavor and nutritional content. Fresh fruits and vegetables are rich in essential vitamins, minerals, and antioxidants that support overall health and well-being.

2. Enhanced Flavor Profiles: Eating in-season means indulging in produce at its freshest and most flavorful state. Ripe tomatoes in the summer, crisp apples in the fall, and tender asparagus in the spring - each season brings its distinct taste sensations.

3. Lower Environmental Impact: By choosing seasonal ingredients, you reduce the demand for out-of-season produce, which often requires long-distance transportation and extensive resources. Supporting local farmers and choosing locally sourced items also minimizes carbon footprints.

4. Cost-Effectiveness: Seasonal produce is often more abundant and less expensive than out-of-season items. Embracing what's in season can lead to cost savings while diversifying your culinary experiences.

5. Connection to Nature: Eating with the seasons fosters a deeper connection with nature's rhythms and cycles. It reminds us of our place in the natural world and encourages gratitude for the gifts of each season.

Practical Tips for Seasonal Meal Planning:

1. Research Seasonal Produce: Familiarize yourself with the fruits, vegetables, and other seasonal ingredients available in your region. Local farmer's markets, community-supported agriculture (CSA) programs, and seasonal produce guides are valuable resources.

2. Create Seasonal Meal Plans: Plan your meals around the seasonal produce you find. Start with the fresh ingredients you have available and build your recipes around them. This encourages creativity and variety in your dishes.

3. Preserve and Freeze: When you encounter an abundance of seasonal ingredients, consider preserving or freezing them for later use. Making sauces, jams, pickles, or freezing fruits and vegetables allows you to enjoy their goodness throughout the year.

4. Try New Recipes: Seasonal meal planning presents an opportunity to try new recipes that showcase the flavors of the season. Experiment with different cooking methods and spice combinations to elevate your dishes.

5. Mix and Match: Don't be afraid to mix and match different seasonal ingredients. Combine fruits in salads or use vegetables in unexpected ways, making the most of what's available in each season.

6. Opt for Local and Sustainable: Support local farmers and producers by choosing locally grown or raised ingredients whenever possible. This not only boosts the local economy but also guarantees the freshest, most nutritious options.

7. Batch Cooking: Utilize batch cooking to save time and effort during busy weeks. Prepare larger portions of seasonal stews, soups, or casseroles and freeze them for quick and satisfying meals later on.

8. Grow Your Own: If you have the space and resources, consider starting a home garden to grow seasonal herbs, fruits, and vegetables. Growing your food fosters a deeper appreciation for the effort and care involved in the process.

9. Seasonal Beverages: Don't forget to incorporate seasonal beverages into your meal planning. Experiment with iced teas, smoothies, or herbal infusions using fruits and herbs in season.

10. Be Flexible: While meal planning is beneficial, remain flexible with your choices. Sometimes, unexpected seasonal ingredients or limited availability may require you to adapt your plan. Embrace the spontaneity of seasonal cooking.

Seasonal Recipes

Below are some delicious seasonal recipes that highlight the flavors of each season:

Spring:

1. **Asparagus and Goat Cheese Tart:** Celebrate the arrival of tender asparagus with a savory tart made with goat cheese, fresh herbs, and a buttery crust.
2. **Strawberry Spinach Salad with Candied Pecans:** This refreshing salad combines sweet strawberries, baby spinach, and crunchy candied pecans, drizzled with a balsamic vinaigrette.
3. **Lemon Herb Roasted Chicken:** A zesty and aromatic roasted chicken infused with lemon, garlic, and spring herbs like rosemary and thyme.

Summer:

1. **Grilled Vegetable Platter:** Create a vibrant array of grilled seasonal vegetables like zucchini, bell peppers, eggplant, and corn, drizzled with a lemon-herb dressing.
2. **Caprese Salad with Heirloom Tomatoes:** A classic summer salad featuring ripe heirloom tomatoes, fresh mozzarella, basil, and balsamic glaze.
3. **Peach and Raspberry Crumble:** Indulge in a delightful dessert made with ripe peaches, juicy raspberries, and a crumbly topping.

Autumn:

1. **Butternut Squash Soup:** A comforting and velvety soup infused with the rich flavors of roasted butternut squash, cinnamon, and nutmeg.
2. **Apple and Gouda Stuffed Pork Chops:** Succulent pork chops filled with a flavorful mixture of sautéed apples, gouda cheese, and herbs.
3. **Pumpkin Spice Granola:** Embrace the essence of autumn with a homemade granola featuring pumpkin seeds, dried cranberries, and warm spices.

Winter:

1. **Roasted Brussels Sprouts with Cranberries and Pecans:** A delightful side dish showcasing the nutty flavors of roasted Brussels sprouts combined with sweet cranberries and crunchy pecans.

2. **Beef and Mushroom Stew:** A hearty and comforting stew made with tender beef, mushrooms, root vegetables, and a rich broth.
3. **Citrus Salad with Winter Greens:** A refreshing salad featuring a medley of citrus fruits paired with winter greens like kale and radicchio, topped with a honey-lime dressing.

WEEKLY MENU TEMPLATES

Template 1: Classic Weekly Menu

Day	Breakfast	Lunch	Dinner	Snack
Monday	Berry Chia Seed Pudding	Grilled Salmon Salad with Lemon Vinaigrette	Hibiscus and Ginger Iced Tea	Almond Butter Energy Balls
Tuesday	Oatmeal Raisin Cookies	Vegan Lentil Loaf with Tomato Glaze	Zucchini Noodles with Avocado Pesto	Baked Sweet Potato Chips
Wednesday	Iced Raspberry Leaf Tea	Hearty Chicken and Vegetable Stew	Spaghetti Squash Pasta with Chunky Tomato Sauce	Spiced Roasted Chickpeas
Thursday	Chia Seed Hydrating Drink	Stuffed Acorn Squash with Wild Rice and Veggies	Black Bean and Corn Tacos	Spiced Roasted Chickpeas
Friday	Lemon Herb Roasted Chicken with Brussels Sprouts	Green Apple and Spinach Smoothie	Baked Cod with Zesty Lemon Sauce	Fresh Squeezed Orange and Carrot Juice
Saturday	Chocolate Avocado Smoothie	Quinoa-Stuffed Bell Peppers	Lentil and Vegetable Curry	Greek Salad Skewers
Sunday	Golden Milk (Turmeric Milk)	Ratatouille with Quinoa	Tofu Pad Thai with Brown Rice Noodles	Apple Slices with Almond Butter

Template 2: Breakfast, Lunch, and Dinner Menu

Day	Breakfast	Lunch	Dinner	Snack
Monday	Berry Chia Seed Pudding	Grilled Salmon Salad with Lemon Vinaigrette	Hibiscus and Ginger Iced Tea	Almond Butter Energy Balls
Tuesday	Oatmeal Raisin Cookies	Vegan Lentil Loaf with Tomato Glaze	Zucchini Noodles with Avocado Pesto	Baked Sweet Potato Chips
Wednesday	Iced Raspberry Leaf Tea	Hearty Chicken and Vegetable Stew	Spaghetti Squash Pasta with Chunky Tomato Sauce	Spiced Roasted Chickpeas
Thursday	Chia Seed Hydrating Drink	Stuffed Acorn Squash with Wild Rice and Veggies	Black Bean and Corn Tacos	Spiced Roasted Chickpeas
Friday	Lemon Herb Roasted Chicken with Brussels Sprouts	Green Apple and Spinach Smoothie	Baked Cod with Zesty Lemon Sauce	Fresh Squeezed Orange and Carrot Juice
Saturday	Chocolate Avocado Smoothie	Quinoa-Stuffed Bell Peppers	Lentil and Vegetable Curry	Greek Salad Skewers
Sunday	Golden Milk (Turmeric Milk)	Ratatouille with Quinoa	Tofu Pad Thai with Brown Rice Noodles	Apple Slices with Almond Butter

Template 3: Family-Friendly Menu

Day	Breakfast	Lunch	Dinner	Snack
Monday	Berry Chia Seed Pudding	Grilled Salmon Salad with Lemon Vinaigrette	Hibiscus and Ginger Iced Tea	Almond Butter Energy Balls
Tuesday	Oatmeal Raisin Cookies	Vegan Lentil Loaf with Tomato Glaze	Zucchini Noodles with Avocado Pesto	Baked Sweet Potato Chips
Wednesday	Iced Raspberry Leaf Tea	Hearty Chicken and Vegetable Stew	Spaghetti Squash Pasta with Chunky Tomato Sauce	Spiced Roasted Chickpeas
Thursday	Chia Seed Hydrating Drink	Stuffed Acorn Squash with Wild Rice and Veggies	Black Bean and Corn Tacos	Spiced Roasted Chickpeas
Friday	Lemon Herb Roasted Chicken with Brussels Sprouts	Green Apple and Spinach Smoothie	Baked Cod with Zesty Lemon Sauce	Fresh Squeezed Orange and Carrot Juice
Saturday	Chocolate Avocado Smoothie	Quinoa-Stuffed Bell Peppers	Lentil and Vegetable Curry	Greek Salad Skewers
Sunday	Golden Milk (Turmeric Milk)	Ratatouille with Quinoa	Tofu Pad Thai with Brown Rice Noodles	Apple Slices with Almond Butter

Template 4: Vegetarian Menu

Day	Breakfast	Lunch	Dinner	Snack
Monday	Berry Chia Seed Pudding	Vegan Lentil Loaf with Tomato Glaze	Zucchini Noodles with Avocado Pesto	Baked Sweet Potato Chips
Tuesday	Oatmeal Raisin Cookies	Stuffed Acorn Squash with Wild Rice and Veggies	Black Bean and Corn Tacos	Spiced Roasted Chickpeas
Wednesday	Iced Raspberry Leaf Tea	Ratatouille with Quinoa	Tofu Pad Thai with Brown Rice Noodles	Apple Slices with Almond Butter
Thursday	Chia Seed Hydrating Drink	Lentil and Vegetable Curry	Greek Salad Skewers	Fresh Squeezed Orange and Carrot Juice
Friday	Lemon Herb Roasted Chicken with Brussels Sprouts	Hibiscus and Ginger Iced Tea	Spaghetti Squash Pasta with Chunky Tomato Sauce	Spiced Roasted Chickpeas
Saturday	Chocolate Avocado Smoothie	Quinoa-Stuffed Bell Peppers	Green Apple and Spinach Smoothie	Almond Butter Energy Balls
Sunday	Golden Milk (Turmeric Milk)	Hearty Chicken and Vegetable Stew	Baked Cod with Zesty Lemon Sauce	Baked Sweet Potato Chips

Template 5: Quick and Easy Meals

Day	Breakfast	Lunch	Dinner	Snack
Monday	Greek Yogurt Parfait with Berries and Granola	Lentil and Sweet Potato Soup	Grilled Tuna Salad with Avocado Salsa	Hummus with Veggie Sticks
Tuesday	Spiced Chickpea Buddha Bowl	Portobello Mushroom Burgers	Cauliflower Fried Rice with Tofu	Spiced Roasted Chickpeas
Wednesday	Lemon and Poppy Seed Muffins	Mediterranean Farro Salad with Feta	Moroccan Chickpea Stew	Almond Butter Energy Balls
Thursday	Black Bean Breakfast Quesadillas	Turmeric-Spiced Cauliflower Stir-Fry	Butternut Squash and Spinach Lasagna	Fresh Squeezed Orange and Carrot Juice
Friday	Green Apple and Spinach Smoothie	Shrimp Avocado Salad with Citrus Dressing	Grilled Steak with Chimichurri Sauce	Greek Salad Skewers
Saturday	Chia Seed Hydrating Drink	Baked Zucchini Fries	Oven-Baked Greek Chicken with Veggies	Baked Sweet Potato Chips
Sunday	Golden Milk (Turmeric Milk)	Low-GI Avocado Toast with Poached Eggs	Mushroom and Spinach Egg Muffins	Apple Slices with Almond Butter

Template 6: Comfort Food Delights

Day	Breakfast	Lunch	Dinner	Snack
Monday	Oatmeal Raisin Cookies	Lentil and Sweet Potato Soup	Stuffed Acorn Squash with Wild Rice and Veggies	Almond Butter Energy Balls
Tuesday	Lemon and Poppy Seed Muffins	Greek-Style Grilled Chicken Wraps	Spinach and Feta Frittata	Baked Sweet Potato Chips
Wednesday	Chia Seed Hydrating Drink	Low-GI Avocado Toast with Poached Eggs	Spaghetti Squash Pasta with Chunky Tomato Sauce	Spiced Roasted Chickpeas
Thursday	Berry Chia Seed Pudding	Turmeric-Spiced Cauliflower Stir-Fry	Butternut Squash and Spinach Lasagna	Fresh Squeezed Orange and Carrot Juice
Friday	Chocolate Avocado Smoothie	Tofu Pad Thai with Brown Rice Noodles	Grilled Tuna Salad with Avocado Salsa	Greek Salad Skewers
Saturday	Iced Raspberry Leaf Tea	Vegan Lentil Loaf with Tomato Glaze	Mushroom and Spinach Egg Muffins	Hummus with Veggie Sticks
Sunday	Golden Milk (Turmeric Milk)	Quinoa-Stuffed Bell Peppers	Moroccan Chickpea Stew	Apple Slices with Almond Butter

Template 7: Light and Fresh Meals

Day	Breakfast	Lunch	Dinner	Snack
Monday	Green Apple and Spinach Smoothie	Lentil and Sweet Potato Soup	Grilled Tuna Salad with Avocado Salsa	Greek Salad Skewers
Tuesday	Lemon and Poppy Seed Muffins	Quinoa-Stuffed Bell Peppers	Mushroom and Spinach Egg Muffins	Hummus with Veggie Sticks
Wednesday	Spiced Chickpea Buddha Bowl	Vegan Lentil Loaf with Tomato Glaze	Butternut Squash and Spinach Lasagna	Fresh Squeezed Orange and Carrot Juice
Thursday	Chia Seed Hydrating Drink	Turmeric-Spiced Cauliflower Stir-Fry	Oven-Baked Greek Chicken with Veggies	Spiced Roasted Chickpeas
Friday	Berry Chia Seed Pudding	Portobello Mushroom Burgers	Cauliflower Fried Rice with Tofu	Almond Butter Energy Balls
Saturday	Iced Raspberry Leaf Tea	Low-GI Avocado Toast with Poached Eggs	Spaghetti Squash Pasta with Chunky Tomato Sauce	Baked Sweet Potato Chips
Sunday	Golden Milk (Turmeric Milk)	Lentil and Vegetable Curry	Moroccan Chickpea Stew	Apple Slices with Almond Butter

Feel free to customize these templates to suit your taste preferences, dietary requirements, and the availability of seasonal ingredients. Happy cooking and meal planning!

CHAPTER 10

LIFESTYLE TIPS
FOR HORMONAL BALANCE

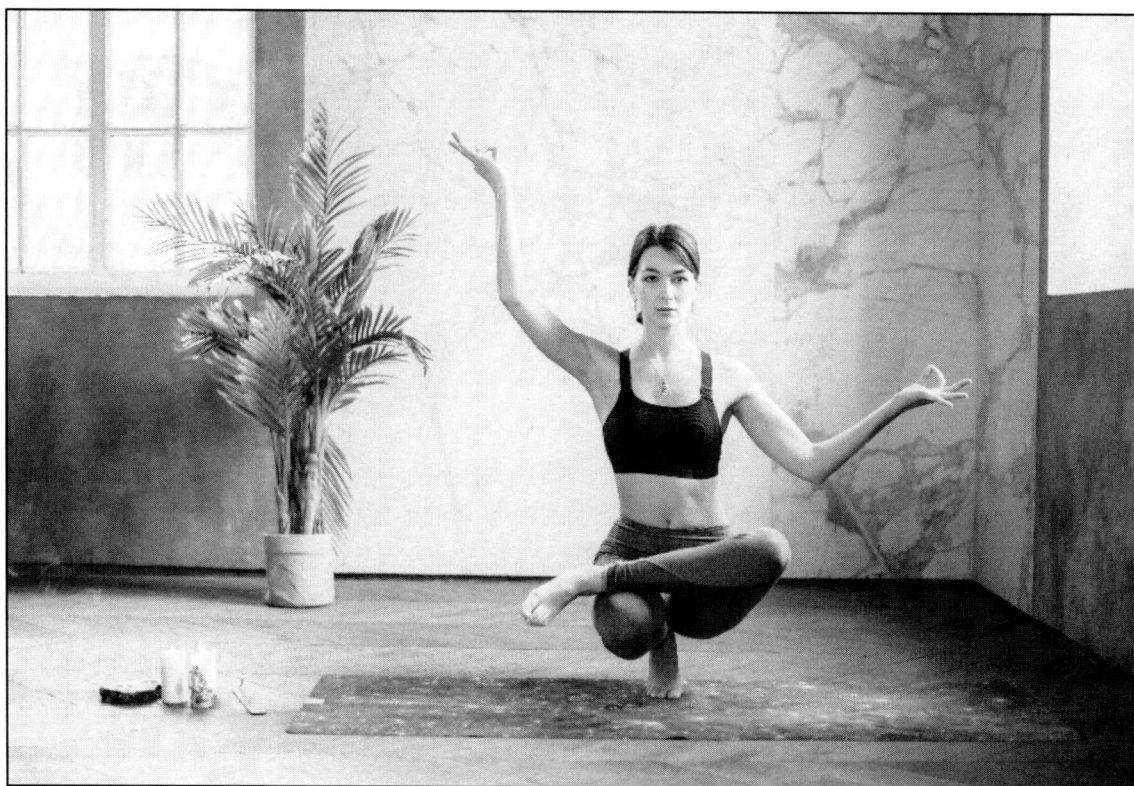

I n this chapter, we will delve into the importance of exercise and physical activity, stress management techniques, sleep optimization strategies, the role of supplements in hormonal balance, and the significance of self-care and mindfulness practices.

EXERCISE AND PHYSICAL ACTIVITY RECOMMENDATIONS

Physical activity is an essential component of maintaining hormonal balance and overall health. Regular exercise can help regulate hormones such as insulin, cortisol, and sex hormones, leading to improved metabolic function and reduced risk of hormonal imbalances. For individuals with conditions such as Polycystic Ovary Syndrome (PCOS), exercise becomes even more crucial, as it can help manage insulin resistance, a common feature of PCOS.

The recommended exercise for hormonal balance includes a combination of aerobic activities, strength training, and flexibility exercises. Aerobic exercises, such as brisk walking, jogging, cycling, or dancing, help improve cardiovascular health and reduce stress levels. Strength training, on the other hand, enhances muscle mass and metabolism, promoting a healthy body composition. Yoga and Pilates, which fall under flexibility exercises, can contribute to stress reduction and relaxation while improving flexibility and balance.

Moreover, finding an exercise routine that one enjoys is essential for adherence and long-term success. Engaging in physical activities that bring joy not only contributes to hormonal balance but also boosts overall well-being and mental health.

STRESS MANAGEMENT TECHNIQUES

Chronic stress can have a profound impact on hormonal balance. When the body is under prolonged stress, it releases excessive amounts of the hormone cortisol, which can disrupt the delicate hormonal equilibrium. Consequently, chronic stress may lead to hormonal imbalances and various health problems, including adrenal fatigue and reproductive issues.

To counteract the negative effects of stress on hormonal balance, incorporating effective stress management techniques into daily life is crucial. Mind-body practices such as meditation, deep breathing exercises, and mindfulness have been shown to reduce stress and promote hormonal balance. Taking time each day to practice these techniques can help individuals cope with stress more effectively and improve their overall hormonal health.

In addition to mind-body practices, engaging in hobbies, spending time in nature, and maintaining a healthy work-life balance can also contribute to stress reduction. Seeking social support and surrounding oneself with positive influences can further enhance one's ability to manage stress and maintain hormonal equilibrium.

SLEEP OPTIMIZATION STRATEGIES

Adequate and restful sleep is vital for hormonal balance and overall health. During sleep, the body undergoes various restorative processes, including hormone regulation and tissue repair. Lack of sleep or poor sleep quality can disrupt these processes, leading to hormonal imbalances and a range of health issues.

To optimize sleep for hormonal balance, several strategies can be adopted. Establishing a consistent sleep schedule, where one goes to bed and wakes up at the same time each day, helps regulate the body's internal clock, promoting better sleep quality. Creating a relaxing bedtime routine, such as reading a book, taking a warm bath, or practicing gentle stretches, can signal the body that it's time to wind down and prepare for sleep.

Additionally, ensuring a comfortable sleep environment with minimal disturbances, such as reducing noise and light exposure, can contribute to better sleep quality. Limiting the consumption of caffeine and electronic devices before bedtime can also aid in falling asleep more easily.

SUPPLEMENTS AND PCOS

Polycystic Ovary Syndrome (PCOS) is a hormonal disorder that affects many women of reproductive age. It is characterized by a range of symptoms, including irregular menstrual cycles, cysts on the ovaries, and hormonal imbalances. While lifestyle changes, such as those mentioned in previous sections, are crucial for managing PCOS, certain supplements have shown promise in supporting hormonal balance and alleviating some of the symptoms associated with this condition.

Inositol

Inositol, a type of B vitamin, has gained attention for its potential benefits in PCOS management. It exists in two forms: Myo-inositol and d-chiro-inositol. Studies have suggested that inositol may improve insulin sensitivity, which is often impaired in women with PCOS. Insulin resistance is a common feature of PCOS and can lead to elevated insulin levels in the blood, contributing to hormonal imbalances and other health issues.

Supplementing with Myo-inositol has been found to help regulate menstrual cycles and improve fertility in women with PCOS. Furthermore, Myo-inositol may reduce the levels of androgens, such as testosterone, which are typically elevated in PCOS. By reducing androgen levels, inositol can help mitigate symptoms like hirsutism (excessive hair growth), acne, and male-pattern hair loss.

Omega-3 Fatty Acids

Omega-3 fatty acids are essential fats that play a crucial role in supporting overall health. They are known for their anti-inflammatory properties, which can be particularly beneficial for individuals with PCOS. Chronic inflammation can exacerbate hormonal imbalances and contribute to insulin resistance.

Some studies have suggested that omega-3 fatty acids may help reduce androgen levels in women with PCOS. By decreasing androgen levels, these healthy fats may contribute to hormonal balance and alleviate symptoms associated with excessive androgens, such as acne and hirsutism.

Moreover, omega-3 fatty acids have been linked to improved heart health, which is particularly relevant for women with PCOS, as they have an increased risk of cardiovascular issues. Incorporating sources of omega-3 fatty acids, such as fatty fish (e.g., salmon, mackerel), flaxseeds, and chia seeds, into the diet can be a beneficial addition to PCOS management.

Vitamin D

Vitamin D, often referred to as the "sunshine vitamin," is crucial for numerous bodily functions, including immune system regulation, bone health, and hormone synthesis. Research has indicated that women with PCOS may have a higher prevalence of vitamin D deficiency compared to women without the condition.

Vitamin D deficiency has been associated with various hormonal disorders, and it may contribute to the development and progression of PCOS. Supplementing with vitamin D has shown promise in improving insulin sensitivity and hormonal balance in women with PCOS.

Additionally, adequate levels of vitamin D have been linked to better mood and mental health, which can be particularly important for individuals with PCOS, as hormonal imbalances can also impact emotions and well-being.

N-acetylcysteine (NAC)

N-acetylcysteine (NAC) is an antioxidant and amino acid precursor that has been investigated for its potential benefits in PCOS management. Oxidative stress, which occurs when there is an imbalance between free radicals and antioxidants in the body, has been linked to hormonal imbalances and insulin resistance in PCOS.

NAC supplementation has been shown to reduce oxidative stress, improve insulin sensitivity, and regulate menstrual cycles in women with PCOS. Furthermore, NAC may help lower androgen levels, which can alleviate symptoms related to excess androgens.

It is crucial to highlight that while these supplements have shown promising results in some studies, they are not a replacement for a balanced diet and healthy lifestyle. Moreover, individual responses to supplements may vary, and it is essential to consult with a healthcare professional before starting any supplementation regimen. A healthcare provider can assess an individual's specific needs, potential interactions with medications, and appropriate dosages to ensure the safe and effective use of supplements in PCOS management.

SELF-CARE AND MINDFULNESS PRACTICES

Self-care and mindfulness practices are essential components of maintaining hormonal balance and overall well-being. In today's fast-paced and demanding world, individuals often neglect their own needs, leading to increased stress and potential hormonal imbalances. Incorporating self-care and mindfulness into daily life can be transformative, promoting a more balanced and fulfilling lifestyle.

Self-Care Practices

Self-care involves deliberately engaging in activities that nurture and support one's physical, emotional, and mental well-being. It is a personalized approach to taking care of oneself, acknowledging that each individual's needs and preferences are unique. Some self-care practices that can contribute to hormonal balance include:

- Hobbies and Creativity: Engaging in hobbies and creative pursuits can be therapeutic and reduce stress. Whether it's painting, writing, gardening, cooking, or playing a musical instrument, dedicating time to activities that bring joy and fulfillment can positively impact hormone regulation.
- Quality Time with Loved Ones: Nurturing meaningful connections with family and friends is essential for emotional well-being. Spending quality time with loved ones, sharing experiences, and offering support can foster feelings of love and belonging, reducing stress hormones and promoting hormonal balance.
- Gratitude and Journaling: Practicing gratitude can shift one's focus towards the positive aspects of life, promoting a more optimistic outlook. Keeping a gratitude journal and regularly reflecting on moments of gratitude can help reduce stress and improve emotional resilience.

- Pampering and Relaxation: Taking time for pampering and relaxation can be rejuvenating and reduce stress levels. Activities like taking a long bath, getting a massage, or simply enjoying a quiet moment with a cup of tea can provide a much-needed escape from the daily hustle and bustle.

- Setting Boundaries: Learning to set boundaries and saying no when necessary can prevent feelings of overwhelm and burnout. Boundaries allow individuals to prioritize their needs and protect their well-being, ultimately contributing to hormonal balance.

Mindfulness Practices

Mindfulness involves being fully present at the moment and observing thoughts and emotions without judgment. It is a practice that can help individuals become more aware of their bodies, emotions, and responses to stress, fostering a deeper understanding of their hormonal health. Mindfulness practices that support hormonal balance include:

- Meditation: Regular meditation practice has been shown to reduce stress, anxiety, and depression. By calming the mind and focusing on the breath or a particular point of focus, meditation can activate the body's relaxation response and counteract the effects of chronic stress on hormonal balance.

- Yoga: Yoga combines physical postures, breathing exercises, and meditation, making it a comprehensive mind-body practice. It can help reduce cortisol levels, lower blood pressure, and improve overall well-being.

- Conscious Consumption: Conscious consumption refers to being entirely present and observant of the sensory details when eating, like the flavor, feel, and scent of your food. This approach can guide individuals towards better food decisions and cultivate a more harmonious connection with their diet, consequently promoting hormonal well-being.

- Nature Walks: Spending time in nature has a calming effect on the mind and body. Going for nature walks or simply spending time outdoors can reduce stress hormones, enhance mood, and improve overall mental health.

- Breathing Exercises: Deep breathing exercises can quickly shift the body from a stress response to a relaxation response. Practicing deep, diaphragmatic breathing activates the parasympathetic nervous system, which promotes relaxation and hormonal balance.

CONCLUSION

As we reach the end of *The PCOS Diet Cookbook*, I hope that you feel empowered, inspired, and equipped with the knowledge and tools you need to manage PCOS effectively. This journey is not just about changing your diet; it's about transforming your lifestyle and embracing a new perspective on health and wellness.

Throughout this book, we have explored the role of nutrition in managing PCOS, delved into the science behind hormonal balance, and discovered the power of food as medicine. We have shared delicious, nourishing recipes designed to support your hormonal health and overall well-being. We have also discussed practical strategies for sustainable lifestyle changes, from meal planning and portion control to exercise, stress management, and sleep optimization.

Remember, managing PCOS is not a sprint; it's a marathon. It's about making small, sustainable changes that add up over time. It's about listening to your body, honoring its needs, and nourishing it with wholesome, nutrient-dense foods. It's about finding balance, not just in your hormones but in all aspects of your life.

As you continue on your journey to hormonal balance, I encourage you to revisit the pages of this book often. Use it as a guide, a reference, and a source of inspiration. Experiment with the recipes, adjust them to your taste and feel free to get creative in the kitchen. Remember, this is your journey, and there's no one-size-fits-all approach to health and wellness.

I am deeply grateful for the opportunity to share my knowledge and passion with you through this book. I hope that it serves as a beacon of hope and a source of empowerment for you and all the women battling PCOS. Remember, you are stronger than PCOS, and with the right tools and knowledge, you can thrive.

Thank you for embarking on this journey with me. Here's to your health, happiness, and hormonal balance. Here's to thriving with PCOS.